eat beautiful

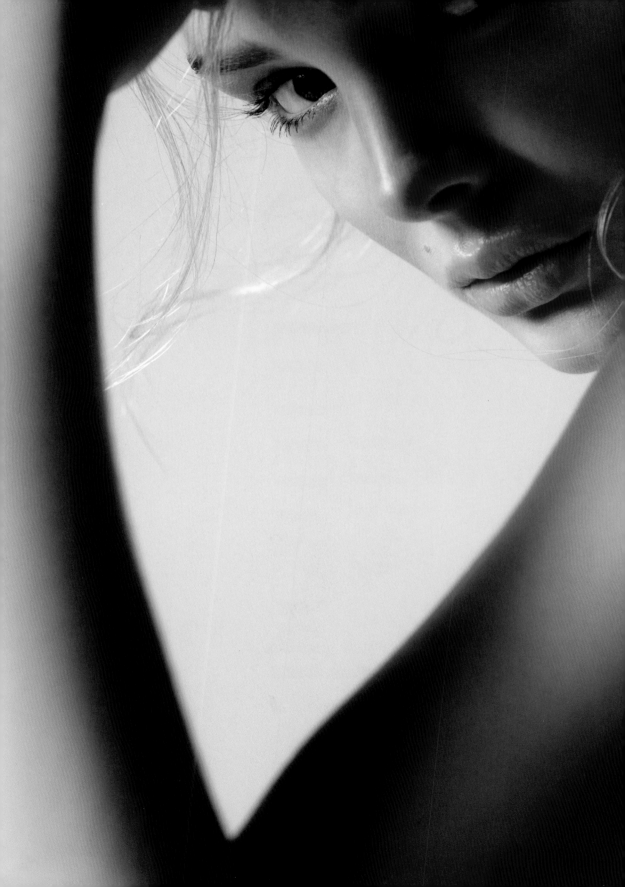

FOOD AND
RECIPES TO
NOURISH
YOUR SKIN
FROM THE
INSIDE OUT

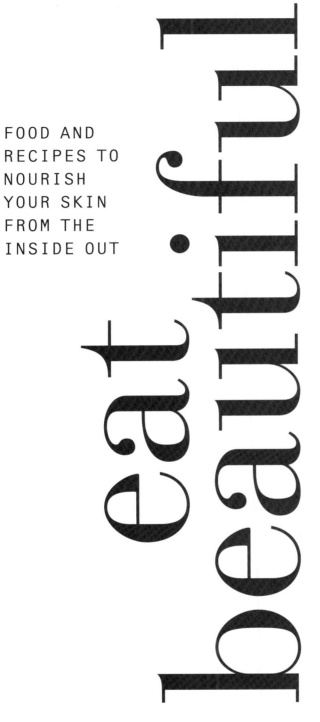

eat·beautiful

WENDY
ROWE

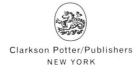

Clarkson Potter/Publishers
NEW YORK

I dedicate this book to my Mum and Dad for allowing me to
be who I am and who always told me to try my best.
To my Mum, for all her creativity and inspiration. To my Dad,
for his motivation and for making every activity an adventure.
Here's my gift to you xxx

Published in the United States by Clarkson Potter/Publishers, an imprint of the Crown Publishing Group, a division of Penguin Random House LLC, New York.
crownpublishing.com
clarksonpotter.com

CLARKSON POTTER is a trademark and POTTER with colophon is a registered trademark of Penguin Random House LLC.

Originally published by Ebury Press, an imprint of Ebury Publishing, a division of Penguin Random House UK, London, in 2016.

Library of Congress Cataloging-in-Publication Data is available.

ISBN 978-0-8041-8958-3
eBook ISBN 978-0-8041-8959-0

Printed in China

Book design: Sandra Zellmer
Food photographs: David Loftus
Beauty photographs: Camilla Akrans
Author photograph: Jem Mitchell
Collage photographs: Camilla Akrans, Jem Mitchell, and Wendy Rowe

10 9 8 7 6

First U.S. Edition

Contents

Foreword by Sienna Miller

I first started working with Wendy in 2007, and she has
done my makeup ever since. Aside from the fact that she
is the most hysterical and fantastic company, I genuinely
believe that there is no one more talented working in
her field. She has a complete artist's ability to understand
light and shade and is a pioneer with skin.

I have often wondered how she managed to look as
fantastic and glowing as she does, while also knowing that
she is on a plane every other week, and this nutritional bible
is the secret! I have tasted Wendy's food and the recipes
are inspiring and delicious – just like the woman herself.

It is so refreshing to find a genuinely informative nutritional
book that is written by someone who is honest, not trying
to preach or inflict guilt, who knows how to have more
fun than anyone and is one of the great women of the world.
It is a gift to us all and I can't wait to get cooking!

Everyone wants
great skin
with a healthy glow.

I f you asked me years ago, I would have said that great skin is mostly due to makeup and skincare. Makeup is my profession, after all, and making people look their best my trade. I've become known as the "master of nudes." Why? Because I figured out a way to do makeup that was invisible to the eye but made the client's skin look amazing and enhanced her features.

But things never stand still, least of all in fashion, and it's been a continuous learning curve since. I've battled my way to the top of my profession, bumbling along with no advice or mentoring, just working things out for myself. I've learned loads and I've learned the hard way – through mistakes and trial and error. I've been put in tricky situations, working with far from perfect skin or in difficult environments. Up a freezing-cold mountain or in a stiflingly hot village in Zanzibar, makeup can react really differently.

When you're a makeup artist, people expect you to know everything, and not just about makeup. I'm not a paramedic, a GP, a psychotherapist or a dermatologist, but when something goes down on a shoot, I'm expected to sort out all problems, from black eyes to broken relationships. I've become good at hiding imperfections, applying skin products as a temporary measure. There is no quick fix to achieve a perfect complexion.

I've become
known
as the "master
of nudes."

Up until recently, we treated the skin from the outside; you would go to the doctor and get a topical cream. But I've come to see that skin troubles are a reflection of what's going on inside. To get perfect skin and maintain it, you need the right balance inside and out. Even top models have problems. They have to deal with problems ASAP – cleaning out their system – after all, they're just like us but it's their job to look good.

While I live and breathe makeup, I believe that beautiful skin comes first – makeup won't look good if the skin is clogged or irritated. And the skin won't look good unless you pay attention to your health in general and your diet in particular. This book is not about makeup, but about how to achieve beautiful skin.

My work as a makeup artist has taken me all around the world. I've learned a lot from other cultures, discovering how traditional approaches to health, food and skincare can really work. It was during my time in Paris (I lived there for 4 years and of course my French is amazing – *not!*) that I found what a difference it makes to use fresh organic produce and eat according to the seasons. If something wasn't in season, you couldn't buy it. This actually helped me to lose weight as it was quality produce.

A seasonal approach underpins this book. I've tried to present foods according to the season in which they are grown, or according to what's best for your health and your skin at a particular time of year. And because looking after your skin on the outside is important, too, I've added a section on skincare, including my routine (a fail-safe approach – but only if you keep it up!) and self-help tips for skin types, plus ideas for making your own beauty aids.

I like to think of stretching as the body smiling, and dancing as the body laughing.

Exercise really helps, too. I have always been active and love the endorphin rush it gives me. The fact that my skin looks so much better for it is an added bonus. The body needs to move; it loves to move. If it doesn't, everything just seizes up and problems arise. Getting your heart rate up and breaking a sweat is key to eliminating toxins. I like to think of stretching as the body smiling, and dancing as the body laughing. Anybody can do these things. Excercise does not have to be regimented; don't get bogged down by the gym!

I must emphasize that I'm not an expert on the subject and I'm not a doctor, though I've worked with a nutritionist on some of the finer details. A lot of what I say in this book is based on common sense and on information I've gathered from simply taking an interest in food and what the nutrients can do for the skin.

*Your body will tell you
what you need,
but it doesn't scream, it whispers,
so try to listen.*

I've tried to break this down so that the dishes are simple and easy to make, with a focus on incredible produce and ingredients chosen for their powers to feed the skin. The all-important thing is to select foods from as wide a range as possible. Your health and skin will definitely benefit; you just need to bear in mind that none of the foods – alone or in combination – are a miracle cure.

I've written this book because I wanted to inspire you to think more about the food you eat and what it can do for your skin, with recipes and beauty tips that are simple and accessible and can easily be integrated into your daily routine. You don't have to do everything – just use it as a springboard for your own ideas. But every little adjustment will help – I promise. I know it's hard and, to be honest, I don't always practice what I preach, especially when I'm pressed for time. On the other hand, I know that when I don't bother, my body tells me about it – I feel bloated, uncomfortable, and my mouth feels sore and my skin is irritated.

Listen to your body, even though it's hard because there's so much going on these days, so much to distract us. Your body will tell you what you need, but it doesn't scream, it whispers, so try to listen. And try to relax and enjoy yourself, too, because the way to achieve that healthy glow is really very simple – just laugh, exercise and feed the skin. A little bit of makeup never hurt any of us either.

Wendy x

beauty
and food

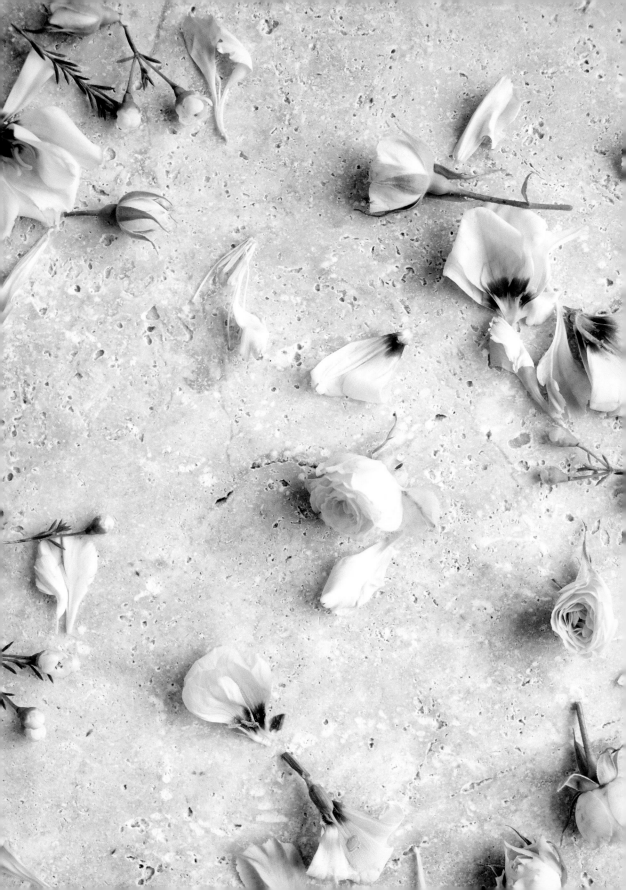

I'm a big believer in nurturing not only the outer skin, but also what lies beneath – our organs and intestines. What's happening in our outer skin – the skin that we can see – is often a reflection of the health of our insides; our organs are hugely hard-working and important in their own right. If you don't service the car, it's not going to work well. Skincare is important, of course, but eating a range of good-quality, skin-friendly foods – seasonal and organically produced when possible – will provide the best foundation. This will ensure your skin has a healthy glow.

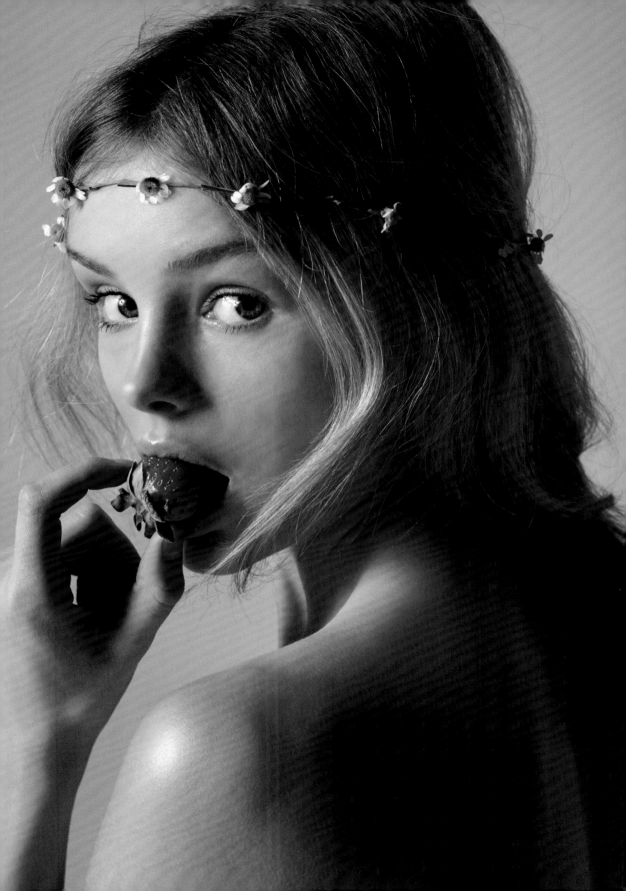

Good digestion

Good skin isn't possible without a well-running digestive system. I know from personal experience that if my digestion is "off," it shows in my skin, which looks dull and is prone to blemishes. It's increasingly apparent that skin disorders are connected to problems in the gut. The root cause of many issues, if you ask a naturopathic doctor, is an overgrowth of candida, a naturally occurring fungus that's present in the intestinal tract. Left unchecked, it's thought that candida can break through the wall of the intestine and get into the bloodstream, releasing toxins that eventually erupt in the skin. The reason we get this overgrowth is down to a number of possible factors, including diet, excessive alcohol consumption, overuse of antibiotics, oral contraceptives and the usual suspect – stress. Above all, candida overgrowth leads to poor digestion, which means you can't absorb the nutrients in the food that you're eating, plus a host of other symptoms (see below). If you think you might be affected, it's best to get checked by a naturopath.

CHECKLIST
FOR SIGNS THAT YOU MIGHT BE SUFFERING FROM CANDIDIASIS

*   Digestive problems: bloating, constipation or diarrhea
*   Tiredness
*   Weight gain
*   Skin issues like eczema, psoriasis or a rash
*   Irritability
*   Strong sugar cravings

PREBIOTICS AND PROBIOTICS

There are ways to naturally claim back control of your gut health, including cutting out the dietary offenders such as refined sugar or alcohol. Making sure you eat plenty of fibrous plant-based foods, to help keep things moving through the intestinal tract, is vital too. When the fiber is non-digestible – as in the case of bananas, for instance, or Jerusalem artichokes – it's known as a "prebiotic," which feeds the good bacteria you already have. Probiotics like "live" yogurt, kefir, or fermented foods such as sauerkraut, miso or tempeh, will help increase the healthy flora in the gut. You can take probiotics in capsule or liquid form, too – available from a good organic chemist or online. Just avoid "probiotic" drinks that are full of sugar. A roughage-rich diet will help your gut to function at its best, making it better able to absorb all those skin-benefiting nutrients to help restore a healthy glow.

INDIGESTION

Even if you're careful about what you eat, it's easy to get indigestion from time to time. No need to pop a pill, though – just try one of these natural remedies:

*   Chew a handful of anise, cardamom pods or fennel seeds.
*   Infuse a few sprigs of fresh peppermint in a cup of water for a few minutes.
*   Add a few slices of fresh ginger to a mug and pour over some hot water to help relieve a stomachache.

Detoxification

A healthy, fully functioning liver is crucial to the body's detoxification process. When the liver is overworked and less able to eliminate toxic waste products, it often shows up in the skin in the form of breakouts and rashes. Our sluggish livers are a product of a modern lifestyle – overburdened by exposure to toxins in the form of alcohol, fatty foods and too much sugar, which need to be constantly filtered out of the system to keep us healthy.

SIGNS THAT YOUR LIVER
MAY NOT BE
WORKING AT ITS BEST

- Bloating
- Itchy and/or blotchy skin
- Acne or rosacea
- Regular acid reflux (heartburn)
- Difficulty losing weight

LUCKILY, THERE ARE VARIOUS
WAYS YOU CAN SUPPORT
THE LIVER SO IT CAN KEEP
YOUR SYSTEM CLEAN AND
YOUR SKIN SUPER HEALTHY

- Start each day with a glass of hot water with a dash of lemon juice.
- Eat lots of fresh veggies.
- Add garlic and turmeric to your meals.
- Choose foods that help the liver function better, such as onions, broccoli, kale, Brussels sprouts, cabbage and cauliflower.
- Take a break from alcohol and caffeine.
- Opt for dandelion tea (see p. 258) or milk thistle tablets/tea.
- Use a tongue scraper in the morning to remove any toxins that have built up overnight (especially after a big night out).

Eat the rainbow

I love eating a plateful of different-colored foods, knowing that it's not just a feast for the eyes but it's doing me so much good at the same time. Eating fresh fruit and vegetables in an array of different colors ensures you're getting the full spectrum of nutrients the body needs to function well. This is all down to particular plant compounds or phytochemicals (see p. 264) with amazing nutritional benefits both for the body and the skin. For example, red fruits and vegetables – such as red peppers, watermelon, tomatoes and certain berries – contain lycopene, a nutrient that helps protect against the damage caused by UV light, and its aging effects on the skin, as well as reducing inflammation and stimulating cell renewal. Orange fruits and vegetables – like carrots, mango and melon – contain the pigment beta-carotene, which the body converts to vitamin A, an incredible resource for the health of both the skin and the eyes. We're forever being told to eat our greens – from kale and spinach to avocados and green beans. And that's absolutely right because they too are a rich source of antioxidant plant compounds – a powerhouse of bio-available beauty helpers. At the indigo end of the rainbow there are all the purple-hued fruit and vegetables – beets, eggplant, cherries, blueberries and black grapes – full of flavonoids that promote heart health and help combat the effects of photo-aging.

Quitting sugar

You may have heard of the disruptive effect refined sugar has on our bodies, causing our energy levels to shoot up and down like a yo-yo and leaving us like junkies looking for the next fix when our blood sugar drops. Did you know that sugar is also a real no-no for the skin? If you consume too much, it damages the collagen and elastin in your skin, making it look dull and more prone to wrinkles. The body stops producing collagen from about the age of 25, after which it will naturally begin to break down over time. Eating too much sugar just accelerates the process. Natural sweeteners can help if you're trying to wean yourself off refined sugar: sugar alternatives like honey and dates not only taste incredible but also help in the quest for beautiful skin.

Healthy oils and fats

Rich in essential fatty acids (see p. 263), good oils are another matter entirely. Bear in mind that not all oils and fats are created equal: it's important to avoid overly processed varieties like canola oil or spreads made with hydrogenated oils, and be mindful of how heat can change the structure of an oil or fat too. I use either raw coconut oil or ghee (see p. 147), both of which don't change their structure at a high heat and both have anti-inflammatory properties. Olive oil and butter are good for use at moderate temperatures, but won't remain stable at a high heat. I love to use flaxseed, macadamia, walnut and extra-virgin olive oils for pouring over dishes such as salads or soups.

Tuning in to the seasons

We're lucky to have access to pretty much any food we want at any time of the year. Food can be imported from anywhere in the world but I do believe that food produced closer to home and in season is better for you. The chances are that the food has been artificially kept "alive" in some facility, possibly with the aid of added chemicals or freezing. This affects not just the flavor, but also the nutrients, with a bonus effect on the health of your skin. I try to follow the principles of Ayurveda, by eating according to the season as much as possible, and by tapping into what's growing where I'm living – it makes good sense, and feels better, too. I love how food changes with the seasons – different fruit and vegetables growing according to when it's hot or cold – and how your body is attuned to wanting those things at the same time. Listen to mother nature.

Avoiding stress

As we age, our ability to recover from the effect of the stress hormone cortisol decreases, and the hormone lingers for longer periods in the body. Stress is toxic for the immune system and has an aging effect, damaging the skin's collagen and natural moisture levels. When stressed, your body also produces adrenaline. Too much adrenaline decreases blood flow and diverts nutrients and oxygen away from the skin, which allows toxins to build up, leading to problems such as breakouts and cellulite.

Stress-busting tips

BREATHE DEEPLY

We often forget this simple act, but increasing oxygen helps us to think more clearly. Focusing on the "in" and "out" breath will clarify thoughts and calm the mind. Make sure to breathe in from the bottom of your stomach before letting your breath out again.

SLEEP IT OFF

Aim for 8 hours' sleep a night. I get impatient if I don't have enough sleep, especially after a long flight when I'm trying to readjust to a new time zone. Try to go to bed at the same time every night to train your body to wind down on cue. Our body is thrown into chaos by disrupted sleep patterns. Lack of sleep takes its toll on the skin, too, as this is when the body has time to regroup and heal itself.

VISUALIZE CALM

Meditating before I go to sleep is really helpful and visualization can be a powerful tool, too. Close your eyes and choose a place – a holiday location or hideaway – or a soothing color. Having a calming image that you can conjure up during stressful times will help train your mind to deflect anxiety.

QUIET THE MIND

Download a mindfulness app to train your mind to be better able to cope with stress and "silence the chatter" of ongoing anxiety.

DO A TECH DETOX

Being constantly "on" and available impacts upon your ability to relax. Making a conscious decision to switch off gives your brain a break from information-processing.

RUN A BATH

It's pretty hard to hold on to stress in a bath. I add a few drops of lavender essential oil to boost relaxation and add to the calming atmosphere. Focus on the good is my mantra.

WORK IT OUT

Getting the blood pumping with a high-intensity short workout will help get the body back into clear-headed order, thanks to the oxygenation and the rush of endorphins. It's hard to think about anything when you are working out.

LISTEN TO MUSIC

Music is a mood changer. Play something that you love – it can really bring you up. To re-energize, put on a track that gets you dancing. And to be peaceful, play something beautiful. Whatever floats your boat.

ENJOY LIFE

Do things that give pleasure or bring peace – cooking, gardening or curling up with a book. See friends and have a laugh whenever you can. Life is short, so have fun!

Mindful eating

Eating should be a pleasure and not something done absentmindedly. Try to be present when you're eating and enjoy the food in front of you. Take your time.

- Sit down at a table.
- Be conscious of your body; don't allow yourself to be all crunched up – your food can't move through your body easily otherwise.
- Don't get distracted by phone calls – you should be enjoying the moment.
- Be conscious of the act of eating.
- Chew each morsel 40 times before swallowing. (I know it sounds a lot, but it does work; even chewing ten times, rather than a hasty couple of bites, makes a difference.) This is said to stimulate your digestive enzymes, which help to break down your food.

- Limit your portion sizes – no more than you can imagine holding in your two hands cupped together – and eat with a smaller fork or spoon to avoid eating too quickly.
- Eat slowly and pay attention to when you're full. It takes at least 15 minutes of eating for the signal to reach your brain that you are full.
- When you eat something that makes you feel bloated, take note and avoid it in the future.
- Notice when something you're eating – e.g., a food or drink containing caffeine or sugar – makes you feel anxious or hyper. What lifts you up will bring you down again with a bump. Try cutting out the food in question to keep on an even keel.
- Notice when your mouth is sticky or you have a headache. You're probably dehydrated and need water first and foremost. (See "Hydration" on p. 249.)

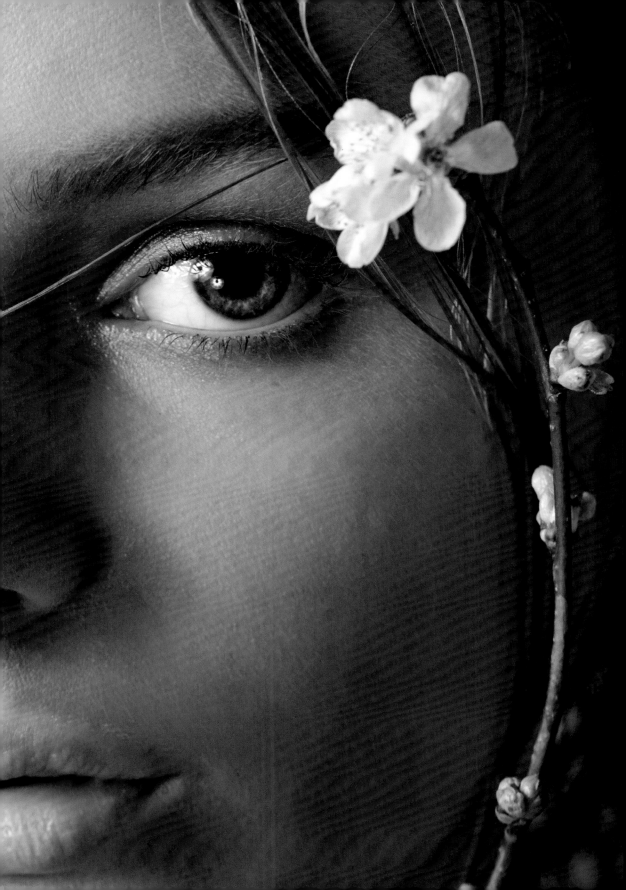

Keep moving

Exercise can do so much more than just keeping you fit. Getting the blood moving through the body is hugely important for restoring a healthy glow or flush of color to the skin. Your body is designed to be constantly on the move, so allowing it to do so helps the blood to circulate, improves oxygenation and speeds the delivery of nutrients to where they're needed. Exercise also works to aid detoxification and lymphatic drainage, which in turn creates that vibrant look of health. And there's nothing like sweating it out if you've got a hangover. You will get rid of toxins much more speedily if your body's moving. When it comes to choosing the type of exercise, do what works for you: yoga is good for stretching tight muscles and for squeezing out the toxins and any pent-up emotion. Sweating for 15–20 minutes a day is a good start. Mix it up because it should always be fun. People tend to forget that dancing is also a form of exercise. Try to approach it so that it is achievable on a weekly basis. Periods of intense exercise can be more harmful and put your body at risk of injury. You're not an athlete, so be realistic – just remember: slowly slowly catchy monkey.

"Wendy is a close friend and we have worked together for a long time. To me, beauty starts with beautiful skin, and Wendy definitely knows how to achieve great skin. She eats super healthy and cooks beautiful food, which I've had the privilege to enjoy. I trust Wendy and any time I have problems with my skin or need a new makeup trick, she's the person I go to for advice. Wendy is a skin and beauty guru!" — **Anja Rubik**, model

Intermittent fasting

Fasting has been used by different cultures for centuries – for cultural and religious reasons, but for the purposes of healing the body and skin, too. Though it's counterintuitive – we've been trained to believe we need three square meals a day to be healthy – fasting can have many positive outcomes for the body. In fact, all of us will have involuntarily fasted at some point: falling ill with a stomach bug forces us to stop eating – and sometimes even drinking – while our body goes into repair mode; and we naturally "fast" through the night, "breaking" it in the morning. Intermittent fasting has a similar effect, allowing the body to redirect its energy from digesting food into repair and detoxification, with the liver and kidneys benefiting especially from the break. Other bodily processes speed up during fasting, making it helpful for addressing problems with the skin, including contact dermatitis, hives, eczema and acne.

The 5:2 diet – consisting of two "fasting" days a week (eating no more than 500 calories a day, which is akin to fasting) and five "normal" days – is wonderfully straightforward in its approach and surprisingly easy to follow once you've got the hang of it. Intermittent fasting is a simple tool we can use whenever we need to "reboot" our system, with quite dramatic results all round. If you switch something on and leave it running without a break, it will soon show signs of wear and tear. Giving your body a break from digestion for a day – even just one day a month – will have a positive impact.

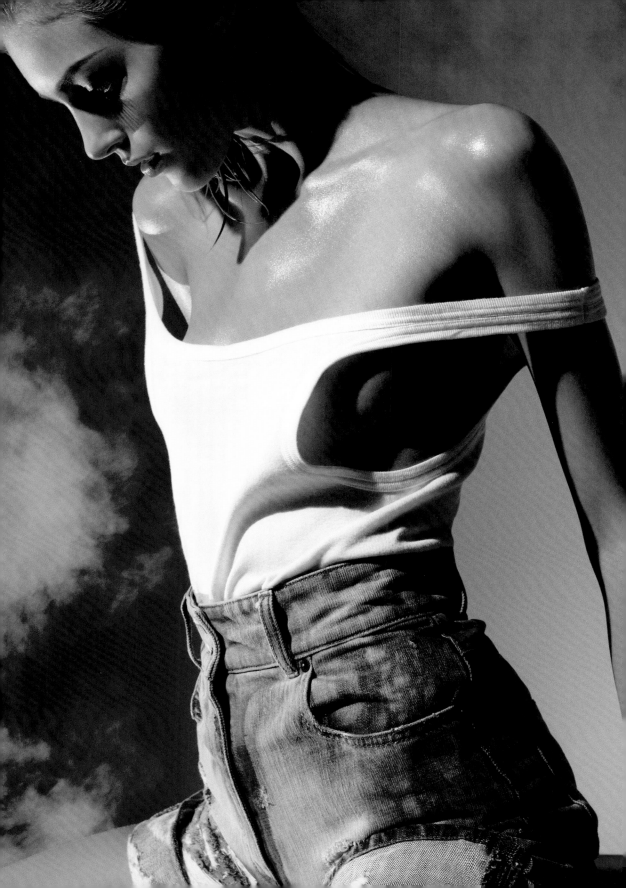

Alcohol

Alcohol is not great for your complexion. It has a high sugar content, which is bad news (p. 16). I think it makes the face look swollen – in fact, it has that effect on the whole body. When I've been overindulging and then stop, my face looks skinnier and gets its structure back. And it's not just me. When I work with celebrities in the summer months – traditionally party time with the booze flowing freely – they say to me, "I'm starting to get the bloated face – help!" Makeup can do a decent camouflage job, but it's better to keep drinking in check.

Don't get me wrong: it's a pleasure to have a glass at the end of the day. Just don't overdo it – your skin will thank you for it!

A GLASS OR TWO ONLY
Don't drink a bottle of wine in one go – it's very easy to do. Try to stick to a glass or two.

ALCOHOL-FREE DAYS
Try to have at least three "dry" days a week.

TEQUILA
I was told about the benefits of drinking tequila by a few celebrities and personal trainers. I was skeptical, but found it actually works. Tequila appears to help with weight loss because of the agavins in it – a form of natural sugar that doesn't raise blood-sugar levels. Many of the calories pass through the system, rather than being absorbed. It has to be clear tequila, not the darker-colored variety. It also stimulates the metabolism and helps dissolve fat. Be careful not to drink too much and remember that it's not a miracle drink. It's still alcohol, which isn't good for you. Drunk in moderation, a good tequila won't give you a hangover. But if you drink cheap tequila, it will knock you for six!

NATURAL WINE
Try drinking natural wine (see p. 197). It is less processed, with no added sugar or chemicals, so it's better for you.

SPIRITS AND MIXERS
A vodka with lime and soda has less sugar than a vodka tonic. Basically, any mixer you put with a clear spirit like gin or vodka is going to up your calorie intake because it's packed with sugar, and you're going to bloat.

BEER AND WINE
They say "never mix the grape with the grain" and they're right – you can get an almighty hangover if you do. If gluten intolerant, avoid grain-based drinks like beer and whisky.

STOUT
Like wine, beer is full of sugar, so drinking several pints will have quite an impact. This is particularly true of stout: downing a pint is the equivalent of eating a pork chop (without the nutrients) – 210 calories in a single pint.

CHAMPAGNE
Sparkling wine is lower in calories than still wine – around 80 per glass, compared to 120 for a glass of red or white. It does go to your head more quickly, of course, making it all too easy to say "yes" to another glass!

FINALLY...
Remember that wine and beer are equally bad for you. You need to do about 20 minutes of hard exercise to work off one glass. One glass of spirits without a mixer can be walked off in about 12 minutes and one alcopop takes roughly 1.5 hours of exercise. I would never drink one of these – it's the processed food of drinks!

Beauty betrayers
and saviors

SOME DOS AND DON'TS TO HELP KEEP YOU HEALTHY AND
YOUR SKIN LOOKING RADIANT

FOOD BETRAYERS

- Refined sugar
- White bread
- Alcohol
- Processed food (anything in a pack)
- Deep-fried food
- Fizzy drinks
- Too much dairy
- Cheap chocolate
- Snacking
- Takeout and fast food
- Margarine
- "Low-fat" anything (yogurt, butter, ice cream, ready meals)
- Dessert on a regular basis

SKIN BETRAYERS

- Alcohol-based toners
- Wearing makeup every day, especially if you have a skin problem (your face needs time to rebalance to avoid congested pores)
- Wearing makeup to the gym (open pores will absorb makeup, becoming clogged)
- Not removing your makeup before bed
- Touching your face unnecessarily (see p. 26)
- Dirty phones
- Looking at your phone or computer just before you go to sleep (see p. 26)

FOOD SAVIORS

- Eating fresh produce, including lots of different-colored fruit and veg (see p. 15)
- Staying hydrated – drink water or coconut water (see p. 249)
- Cooking and eating a leisurely meal
- Eating a light meal in the evening

SKIN SAVIORS

- Following my Non-negotiable Skincare Routine (see p. 246)
- Moisturizing your body and your feet once a day after bathing
- Using a hand cream when your hands are feeling dry
- Spending time outside
- Following my Stress-Busting Tips (see p. 17)
- Having a good chat or doing some meditation; you need to get out what you're thinking – don't hold on to bad emotions
- Trying to achieve at least one thing a day that will make your life easier
- Trying to do one good deed a week
- Doing something creative to improve your mood
- Having a go at something completely different
- Not being a slob – make your bed!

Beauty store cupboard

KITCHEN CUPBOARD AND FRIDGE

- Avocados
- Lemons
- Garlic
- Onions
- Root vegetables (e.g., beet)
- Leafy greens (e.g., kale, spinach)
- Broccoli
- Arugula
- Fresh herbs (e.g., basil, mint, rosemary)
- Fresh ginger
- Eggs
- Oily fish
- Wheat-free crackers
- Buckwheat flour
- Flaxseed flakes
- Dried crushed red pepper flakes
- Miso paste
- Turmeric (fresh root and ground)
- Cayenne pepper
- Cumin (ground)
- Coconut oil
- Olive oil
- Flaxseed oil
- Molasses
- Honey
- Bottles of mineral water
- Mineral and vitamin supplements

BATHROOM CABINET

- Face cleaner
- Moisturizers
- Toners
- Different face masks
- Lip balm
- Hand and foot creams
- Body creams
- Body scrub
- Skin antiseptic
- Epsom bath salts (see p. 243)
- Magnesium spray or cream
- Essential oils (e.g., chamomile, lavender)
- Tiger balm
- Hair spray
- Dry and standard shampoos
- Conditioners
- Tweezers and nail file
- Nail scissors and clippers
- Cuticle trimmers
- Foot buffer
- Razors
- Candles
- Eye cream
- Eye drops

"What separates Wendy is not only her genuine, fun and kind-hearted spirit – it's the fact that she is a visionary and knows about makeup, skincare and health. She is one of the few people who knows how to work with every skin tone." — **Neelam Gill,** model

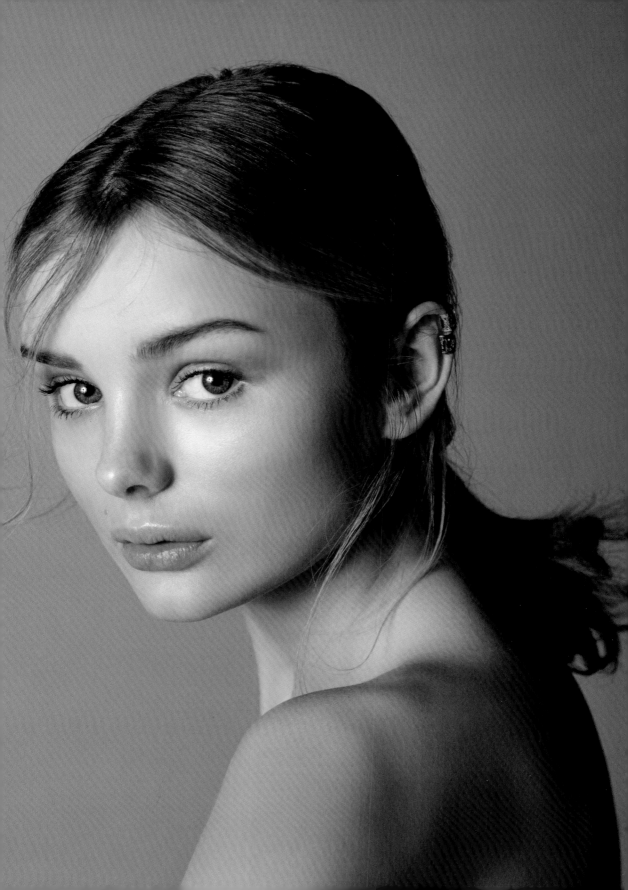

Wendy's golden rules

"BREAKFAST LIKE A KING,
LUNCH LIKE A PRINCE
AND DINNER LIKE A PAUPER"

I collect little pearls of wisdom
like these that help me
to make better lifestyle decisions.

NO RAW AFTER FOUR
Working on the principle that raw foods are harder for the body to break down, it's best to give them time to be digested. Only eat raw before 4pm, when your metabolism is fired up and the stomach is better equipped to digest foods. Some say that raw food prepared properly (soaked, etc.) is fine in the evening, but I stick with salads for lunch and cooked food for dinner.

CHEW, CHEW, CHEW
You need to chew your food to stimulate the enzymes that start breaking down food. If you don't chew enough – at least 40 times – you don't stimulate them sufficiently. The harder it is to break down, the more digestive juices it will need, which is more work for the body.

PURE AND TRUE
If an ingredient is changed fundamentally, avoid it. Steer clear of processed foods, which lose their nutritional value when heat processed or contain chemical additives.

EAT YOUR WATER
It's important to stay hydrated (see p. 249). So drink up your water, and eat it too: foods with a high water content are as effective. Drink up, eat up and restore your glow!

DON'T DRINK YOUR CALORIES
Fruit juices may be pure but they are also high in natural sugars. Bottled smoothies are even worse: they are packed with sugar and low in nutrients, so high in empty calories.

FAT AIN'T BAD
Good fats don't make you fat – sugar does. For too long we've been told that fat is bad and "low-fat" alternatives are better when in fact they're often stuffed with aging and fattening hidden sugars. Look at labels – be sure to avoid sugar-laden foods and don't be scared of good fats (see p. 16).

LISTEN TO YOUR BODY
Your body is a miracle of nature – listen to it. All too often the warning signs are ignored, so that a problem becomes chronic. If you have indigestion after eating a particular food, then avoid it for a while – even keep a food diary to help you to spot a pattern.

HANDS OFF!
I don't want to get all germophobic on you, but please remember to stop touching your face mindlessly. Hands can be filthy things, transferring dirt and acne-causing bacteria from place to place. Clean hands will help keep your skin clear and congestion-free.

EAT LESS AND EXERCISE MORE
Losing a bit of weight is great and feels like a real achievement, but it's so easy to fall into old habits. The key to losing weight and keeping it off is simple: eat less, go to bed early and exercise.

TECH-FREE DIET
It's not good to have electronic devices on all the time, especially just before bed. The bluish light they emit will disturb your sleep.

LIVE AND LET LIVE
The most important rule is to concentrate on **you** and do what feels right for your body.

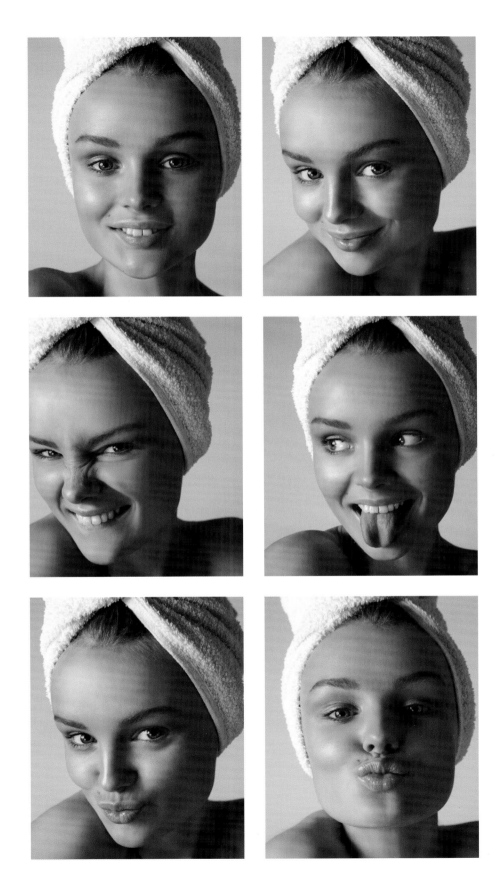

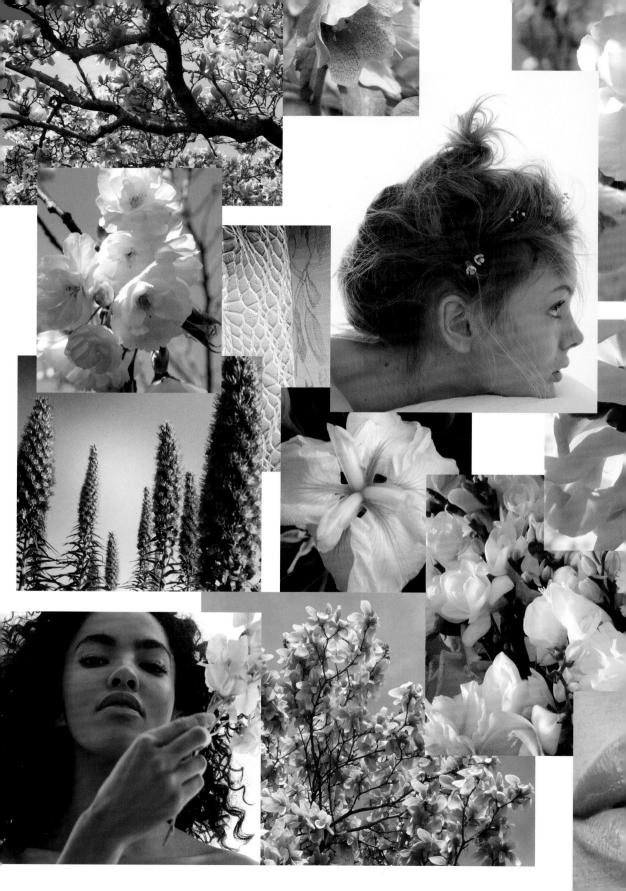

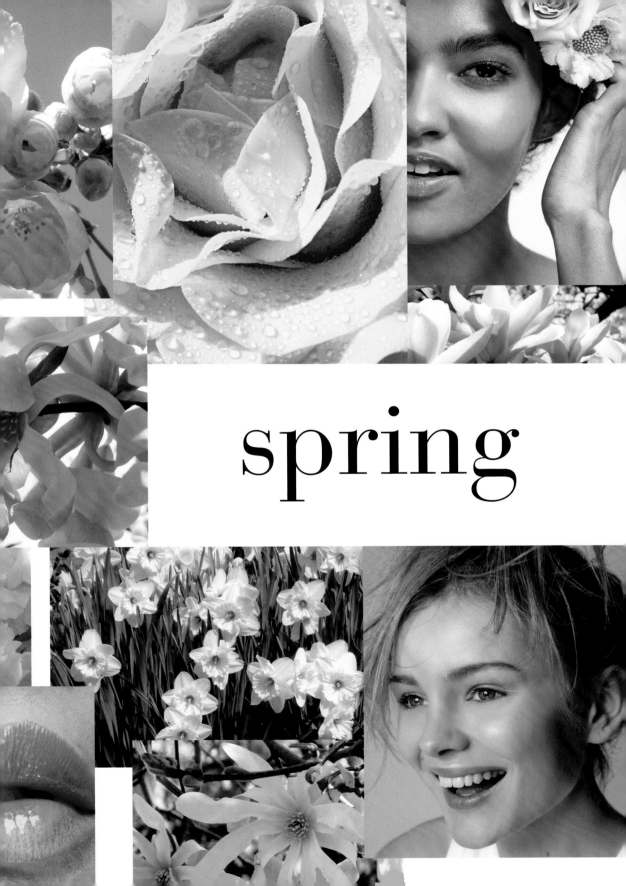

spring

The spring clean

After the back-to-back fashion shoots and shows from mid-October to March, things let up in the spring and I have time to breathe. There's always a sense of optimism when the signs of spring emerge – it's like nature's reward after the hardships of a long winter. Days lengthen, there's more sunlight and I feel more positive. Spring is the season of creativity and new beginnings and skin should be full of new life too: the complexion needs a reboot to restore its natural radiance.

For some, spring can bring irritation, inflammation and breakouts – eczema due to allergies like hay fever can make skin extra sensitive. I find that skin can look dull and dry after the ravages of winter, and in need of rejuvenation and exfoliation. To speed up my skin's recovery, I exfoliate and opt for replenishing and purifying masks during my downtime. Don't overdo it.

Now's the time to start thinking about your bikini body, so that when summer comes around you feel good about yourself. Starting in the spring gives you time to ramp up your exercise routine gradually. This also increases circulation in the body, helping to clear out any toxins left over from winter.

I avoid richer foods like red meat and dairy, and instead go for lots of green vegetables and leaves, along with lighter proteins. Although the science is not definitive, I have a teaspoon of manuka honey with breakfast as I've found that it helps keep allergies at bay.

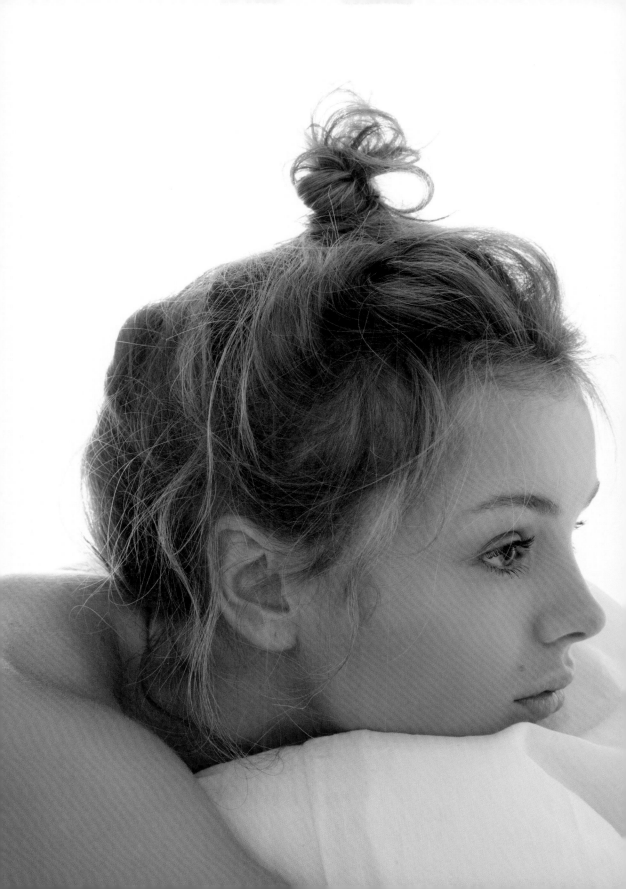

THE SKIN-FRIENDLY ALTERNATIVE TO DAIRY

ALMOND MILK

I've never been a big fan of milk – even when I was a kid. Growing up in the UK, we were made to drink milk at school and I absolutely hated it. When they asked us if we wanted extra milk, my reaction would be "yuck!" Perhaps a telltale sign that my body didn't really need it. Cow's milk is very nutritious, but it's not for everyone. While it's fine to drink it in moderation, some people find that too much can have a negative impact on their well-being. Cow's milk and dairy products in general can be bad for your skin, too, hence cutting them out of your diet can make a big difference if you suffer from skin problems. If you do drink milk, then go for organic to avoid the hormones in standard cow's milk that can be an issue if you suffer from acne. For me, nut milks are the obvious alternative – and almond is my favorite. It is packed with nutrients that work harder for your skin than dairy does. Low in fat but high in energy-giving protein and fatty acids, almond milk also contains calcium, which most people think they have to get from cow's milk, along with numerous other minerals and vitamins. This is nutritionally so much better for the skin, as it not only avoids all the acne-causing inflammation, but actually works to feed the skin as you drink it, helping to keep you feeling full, too, thanks to the fiber content. Homemade almond milk – which you can make by blending a handful of ground almonds with water – tends to be more nutritious, but you can buy it ready-made, too. If you do buy it, make sure you look for organic unsweetened varieties, as it can often include unnecessary sugars, which can irritate the gut and have an aging effect on the skin (see p. 16).

SKIN-FEEDING NUTRIENTS

- Dietary fiber
- Fatty acids
- Minerals:
  calcium
  iron
  magnesium
  phosphorus
  potassium
  zinc
- Protein

- Vitamins:
  A
  B1 (thiamine)
  B2 (riboflavin)
  B3 (niacin)
  B6 (pyridoxine)
  B9 (folate)
  C
  D
  E

ALMOND CHOCOLATE MILKSHAKE (P. 66)

THE MOOD BOOSTER

ARUGULA

I like really dark green vegetables or salad leaves because I know they are high in vitamins and nutrients that help the body in so many ways. I love the peppery flavor of arugula in particular and the fact that you can use it raw to accompany so many different dishes – it goes with just about everything. It is a great mood booster, containing other nutrients that help cleanse the blood and detoxify the system. It is also high in potassium, which improves cardiovascular health, and vitamin K that supports bone health. But more than this, arugula is high in vitamin C, which helps the body produce collagen and fight the impact of free radicals. To get the most vitamin C out of arugula, it is best eaten raw.

SKIN-FEEDING NUTRIENTS

- Dietary fiber
- Minerals:
  calcium
  manganese
  potassium
- Phytochemicals
- Vitamins
  B9 (folate)
  C
  K

ASPARAGUS

THE DETOXIFIER

Eating asparagus is said to make your pee smell, but that's actually a good thing – a sign that the toxins are being flushed out of your system. Any odor is a small downside for a big benefit, you could say. A classic spring vegetable, asparagus is best when it's picked fresh and cooked simply. It's one of those ingredients that's hard to get wrong, plus it's supremely good for you. For a start, asparagus is rich in vitamins and minerals, which makes it excellent for the skin and health in general. It's known to help keep skin clear and youthful-looking, hair and nails strong and the brain functioning properly to promote mental agility – perfect for the scatterbrained! I've already touched on the diuretic properties of the plant, the way in which it helps to flush toxins from the body – especially the liver, which can have a negative impact on the skin when it's suffering from toxic overload. Believed to slow down the symptoms of aging in the skin, asparagus works to nourish from within, also helping to prevent psoriasis, skin dryness and acne. A source of plant-based protein and full of fiber, while very low in calories and carbohydrate, it makes a great choice for anyone trying to lose weight, as it keeps you feeling fuller for longer.

SKIN-FEEDING NUTRIENTS

- Dietary fiber
- Minerals:
  calcium
  copper
  iron
  manganese
  selenium
  phosphorus
  potassium
  selenium
  silica
  zinc
- Phytochemicals:
  carotenoids (beta-
    carotene lycopene)
- Protein
- Vitamins:
  A
  B1 (thiamine)
  B2 (riboflavin)
  B5 (pantothenic acid)
  B6 (pyridoxine)
  B9 (folate)
  C
  E
  K

THE ANTIBACTERIAL SUPERFOOD

B ASIL

I love basil and like to have a plant at home for a source of fresh leaves, to add to dishes or to apply to the skin (see p. 256). The smell of basil always reminds me of Italy, though in fact it probably originated in India, where it has been grown for over five thousand years, and was brought to the Mediterranean via the spice routes in ancient times. There are many different types of basil, from the famed sweet Genoese variety, grown in Liguria in Italy, to Thai basil, which is used a lot in Asian cooking. The taste varies depending on the type of basil, but the nutritional values are the same, with anti-aging properties that make it extremely good for the skin. Rich in antioxidant flavonoids and vitamins, basil fights the aging effect of free radicals in the body, thereby helping to preserve the youthful glow in the skin. The compounds in basil are naturally antimicrobial in their effect, helping restore microbial balance in the gut, with antibacterial properties that make the herb excellent for fighting disease-causing bacteria and hence treating skin conditions such as rosacea and acne.

SKIN-FEEDING NUTRIENTS

- Dietary fiber
- Minerals:
  calcium
  iron
  magnesium
  potassium
- Phytochemicals:
  flavonoids
    (anthocyanin,
    orientin,
    vicenin)
- Vitamins:
  A
  B9 (folate)
  C
  K

B EET

I know I'm encouraging you to be healthy, but I don't expect you to be complete angels. Sometimes we all overindulge a little and wake up feeling somewhat the worse for wear and desperate to get back to normal. Did you know that beet can be your saving grace? This is because it contains nutrients – specifically betalains, responsible for the deep red color – that boost the functions of the liver. The liver is vital for the health of the skin; in fact both the skin and the liver work to detoxify the body, so how they interact with each other is crucial and can't be overestimated. As I've mentioned earlier (see p. 15), the skin can become a dumping ground for any toxins that the body isn't able to eliminate through its usual pathways of the liver and kidneys. You may well have discovered this already after a big night of drinking, when the skin can become inflamed, congested or overly sensitive. Beet has been used for centuries for its liver-healing powers and to help rid the body of toxins. Detoxification is so important for the skin, helping to reduce congestion and inflammation. Beet contains pectin – a form of soluble fiber, which further helps to flush the system, and gives the lymphatic system a natural kick-start, too. Rich in vitamins and minerals, beet also helps support collagen production, so essential to elasticity of the skin.

SKIN-FEEDING NUTRIENTS

- Dietary fiber:
  pectin
- Minerals:
  iron
  manganese
  potassium

- Phytochemicals:
  betalain
  carotenoids
     (beta-carotene,
     lycopene,
     zeaxanthin)
  glutathione
- Vitamins:
  C
  K

BEET AND QUINOA BURGERS (P. 72)

BLUEBERRY

These small berries have more power in them than you think, which is why you see them in so many healthy dishes. No skin-feeding regimen is complete without a regular serving of blueberries, though don't overdo it with them – no more than a handful at a time – as they contain a lot of natural sugar. Small but powerful, they are packed with flavonoids that act as an antioxidant in the body and other nutrients that help keep your skin looking radiant and youthful. They're a rich source of vitamin C, which boosts collagen and skin elasticity. They're even known to help treat the skin by strengthening damaged blood vessels, which should improve broken capillaries, and to improve skin conditions such as rosacea thanks to their powerful anti-inflammatory properties. This berry is also known for its power to support connective tissue further, helping the skin to look firm and taut.

SKIN-FEEDING NUTRIENTS

- Dietary fiber
- Phytochemicals:
  flavonoids
    (anthocyanin)
- Vitamins:
  C

CILANTRO

Like most herbs, cilantro is truly wonderful for treating the skin and wider health. Just remember: if it's green, it's good – packed with nutrients, in fact. Particularly useful in regulating blood sugar, cilantro is terrific at keeping the system on an even keel, which is so helpful in avoiding the inevitable breakouts that follow from blood-sugar spikes – a great herb for any diabetic or acne-sufferer for this reason. Rich in antioxidants, cilantro treats skin with its free-radical-destroying properties, which work to brighten and target signs of aging. It's also a potent antibacterial, antiseptic, antifungal and anti-inflammatory herb – a lot of "antis" that amount to a big plus for the health of the skin, especially in the treatment of serious skin conditions and infections like rosacea, and almost any skin issue that stems from inner inflammation (as most do). A digestive aid, cilantro assists in the production of digestive enzymes, thus preventing excess gas and nausea due to poor digestion – and as we know, a healthy gut equals a healthy-looking complexion. The liver, too, is supported by cilantro, thanks to the presence of potent antioxidants like quercetin, helping it in its function of detoxifying the body.

SKIN-FEEDING NUTRIENTS

- Dietary fiber
- Minerals:
  potassium
- Phytochemicals:
  flavonoids
    (quercetin)
- Vitamins:
  A
  C
  K

CILANTRO AND BEET SALAD WITH
AVOCADO AND MINT (P. 60)

E_{GG}

THE PERFECT PROTEIN

Eggs are such a great breakfast food: you can cook them in so many different ways – poached, scrambled, boiled – and they're packed with protein, making them the perfect food to start the day. I'd always assumed that you shouldn't eat too many because they clog up the system. Not true. Did you know that, aside from their protein content, the common egg is also a nutritional powerhouse? The yellow and the white parts of the egg each contain different vitamins and minerals. A lot of people are big on eating just the whites, to avoid the fat content of the yolk, but the yolk is actually packed with nutrients like vitamins A and D, which help to regulate cell turnover in the skin, while the nutrients in egg whites work to repair and brighten the skin, too. Eggs are regarded as a "complete" source of protein, as they contain all nine essential amino acids (these are the ones we can't produce, and must obtain from our diet), making them really important to include in the diet for this reason alone. Go for organic or free-range eggs whenever possible: because they have higher levels of skin-benefiting omega-3 fatty acids and to avoid the chemical additives fed to intensively farmed chickens. Eggs from happier, more ethically reared chickens taste better too – I certainly feel better eating them.

SKIN-FEEDING NUTRIENTS

- Fatty acids:
  omega-3
- Minerals:
  copper
  iron
  lecithin
  selenium
  zinc
- Protein:
  all nine essential
    amino acids

- Vitamins:
  A
  B2 (riboflavin)
  B6 (pyridoxine)
  B12 (cobalamin)
  D
  E
  K

SKIN-FRIENDLY FRITTATA WITH
SALSA VERDE (P. 54)

EGGPLANT

Going by the intense, dark purple shade of the eggplant, you can be sure it's a vegetable that's abundant in skin-beautifying antioxidants. A member of the nightshade family of vegetables – so named because they often prefer to grow in the shade or at night – eggplant contains flavonoids whose antioxidant properties help counteract the signs of aging as well as promote heart health. One particular flavonoid – nasunin – works to protect skin cells from damage, transports nutrients like iron around the body while also working to eliminate toxins from the system. It's important to eat the skin of eggplant because that is where the nutrients that help to improve blood circulation are stored. The skin also has an anti-inflammatory effect on the body, making it an excellent choice for a complexion-repairing diet. Low in fat and carbohydrates but high in fiber, the eggplant is the perfect basis for a healthy meal: not only will it fill you up, but it will feed your skin and body with its rich load of minerals, vitamins and other nutrients.

SKIN-FEEDING NUTRIENTS

- Dietary fiber
- Minerals:
  calcium
  iron
- Phytochemicals:
  flavonoids
    (nasunin)

- Vitamins:
  A
  B1 (thiamine)
  B2 (riboflavin)
  C
  D
  E

LEAFY GREENS

Whenever I eat a meal, I start to panic if there are no leafy greens, because I know how good they are for me and for my skin in particular. An incredibly rich source of vitamins, minerals and age-fighting phytochemicals, dark leafy greens – by which I mean leaves like chard, arugula, kale and spinach – help to beautify in a way that most skincare creams can't. Going straight to the source, the nutrients in greens help support new growth, cell repair and detoxification of the body, so the skin (and hair, nails and teeth) look healthier, stronger and younger. Leafy greens are loaded with vitamin A, which can help treat acne by limiting the production of sebum, and also by helping the system to eliminate toxins for a clearer, calmer complexion. Vitamin E protects the skin from free-radical damage, while folate helps the skin to repair itself and to create new cells. Beta-carotene performs a similar function of protection and cellular renewal, while biotin can speed up cell repair and lutein boosts hydration – all essential at the end of a long summer in the sun. Leafy greens also contain omega-3 fatty acids, which help to maintain healthy cell membranes and keep the skin soft and supple – particularly useful if you're vegetarian and don't eat oily fish.

SKIN-FEEDING NUTRIENTS

- Dietary fiber
- Fatty acids:
  omega-3
- Minerals:
  iron
  magnesium
  potassium
- Phytochemicals:
  carotenoids
    (beta-carotene,
    lutein)
- Vitamins:
  A
  B7 (biotin)
  B9 (folate)
  C
  E

THE SELENIUM-RICH SKIN SAVER

PEARL BARLEY

Like eggs, pearl barley is a complete form of protein, containing all nine amino acids, which you can only obtain from your diet. So if you're not keen on eggs – and I know loads of people who aren't – then pearl barley makes a great alternative. It's a bit of an unsung skin-feeding hero, in my opinion; it doesn't get much press but pearl barley is a hearty grain that's really effective in treating skin conditions. Anti-inflammatory in nature, it's rich in dietary fiber and works to aid digestion, keeping the colon clear – and the skin too as a result. Full of B-complex vitamins and minerals such as iron, calcium, potassium and zinc, quite apart from all those amino acids, pearl barley is a highly nutritious and filling food source that benefits the skin as well as the rest of the body. But I think it's the selenium content in particular that makes pearl barley so effective for the health of the skin. Not only does this help to preserve elasticity, it also protects against UV damage and may help to reverse existing damage, too, making foods rich in selenium an invaluable part of a skin-shielding diet.

SKIN-FEEDING NUTRIENTS

- Dietary fiber
- Minerals:
  calcium
  copper
  iron
  magnesium
  phosphorus
  selenium
  zinc
- Protein:
  all nine essential
    amino acids
- Vitamins:
  B complex

POMEGRANATE

The pretty, jewel-like seeds of the pomegranate have been prized for thousands of years for their nutritional value. Outside of the Middle East, however, it's easy to forget about the pomegranate – not many people think of this exotic fruit as a staple – but it's worth including it as a regular on your shopping list, thanks to its many and varied anti-aging benefits for the skin. Packed with our number-one skin beautifier – vitamin C – pomegranates are known for their ability to stimulate collagen production in the body, which, as we've seen (see p. 251), is hugely helpful in keeping the skin looking taut, young and radiant. Rich in powerful actives that have been shown to preserve collagen and protect against free-radical damage, pomegranates boost elasticity and stimulate collagen-producing cells, helping to reduce wrinkles and sagging skin. They're known to help repair damaged skin and combat inflammation, too, making pomegranates an excellent ingredient in an acne-treatment diet. As you might imagine, the fibrous seeds are brilliant at aiding detoxification – helping the gut to eliminate waste for a clearer colon and more vibrant-looking skin. And as pomegranate seeds are so small, eating them promotes chewing, which in turn stimulates the enzymes in your mouth and your stomach so they are able to break down your food more easily, promoting better digestion. (See p. 18 for more on the benefits of mindful eating.)

SKIN-FEEDING NUTRIENTS

- Dietary fiber
- Minerals:
  calcium
  copper
  iron
  magnesium
  manganese
  phosphorus
  potassium
  selenium
  zinc
- Phytochemicals:
  flavonoids
    (ellagic acid)
  polyphenols
    (punicalagin)

- Vitamins:
  B1 (thiamine)
  B2 (riboflavin)
  B3 (niacin)
  B5 (pantothenic acid)
  B6 (pyridoxine)
  B9 (folate)
  choline
  C
  E
  K

POPCORN

It's hard to imagine, but people have been eating corn for the past six thousand years or so and across different cultures. Simply adding kernels to a heat source would have given our ancestors the fun, popped-corn snack we still eat today. I'm a big fan of popcorn – for me its simplicity is its biggest selling point. A low-cal, gluten-free whole grain, homemade popcorn is also packed full of nutrients – the perfect snack. (However, you need to check the label on shop-bought and never buy popcorn at the movies – it is full of calories!) Loaded with fiber, which of course helps you to feel fuller for longer, staving off those sugar cravings, popcorn actually contains more protein per ounce than potato chips, and a whole lot less saturated fat and empty calories, too. For the skin, popcorn provides nutrients that help to keep it clear and bright, including vitamin B1 (thiamine), which aids circulation and helps the flow of nutrients and waste to and from the skin to promote a healthy glow.

SKIN-FEEDING NUTRIENTS

- Dietary fiber
- Minerals:
  magnesium
  manganese
  phosphorus
  zinc

- Phytochemicals:
  phenolic acids
- Protein
- Vitamins:
  B1 (thiamine)
  B3 (niacin)
  B6 (pyridoxine)
  B9 (folate)

                   SAVORY POPCORN (P. 76)

QUINOA

THE PROTEIN-LADEN POWERHOUSE

I can't remember when or how I was introduced to quinoa – it seemed to come out of nowhere. At first I had no idea how to pronounce it: kwin-o-a, keen-o-a, kween-o-ah? Eventually someone set me straight (keen-wah) and I discovered that, while it's not a grain like wheat and other "true" cereals, it can be used in a similar way and with the advantage of being entirely gluten-free. As soon as I realized it was high in protein and low in carbs – a lot less than in pasta or rice, for instance – it became one of my best food friends. Quinoa is a good source of amino acids, which are great for healing wounds and repairing skin cells, plus it's high in fiber, so it keeps your metabolism moving and your skin clearer as a result – all helped by a good dose of B vitamins for improved skin elasticity and a youthful complexion. So all in all, a no-brainer for me – plus it's super filling so you don't end up stuffing your face with chocolate afterward!

SKIN-FEEDING NUTRIENTS

- Dietary fiber
- Minerals:
  iron
  magnesium
  manganese
  zinc
- Protein:
  amino acids
    (lysine)
- Vitamins:
  B2 (riboflavin)
  B6 (pyridoxine)
  B12 (cobalamin)

RADISH

I enjoy foods that are quite peppery, and radishes make a lovely snack just as they are – I like to have a bowl of them on the kitchen table. They're quite addictive and I always end up eating loads – much better, though, than having a bowl of chips on hand, which are all too easy to hoover up in one sitting. Radishes are high in vitamin C and so have an antioxidant function that helps to restore radiance and build collagen for a clearer complexion. Full of other vitamins as well, radishes help to repair skin damage and to prevent skin disorders – they're a great addition to the diet for anyone with acne or eczema, for instance, as their general anti-inflammatory properties help to calm the skin and restore balance to it. Assisting too with cell replenishment, radishes can bring a "newness" to the skin as they help skin cells turn over. The best time to eat them is when they're naturally in season at the start of spring. The perfect antidote to the dulling effects of a long, cold winter, when our skin is exposed to constant heating and extreme weather conditions, they help to restore radiance for the new season ahead. Working to carry oxygen around the blood, and to control blood-sugar levels, the nutrients in radishes also help to re-establish equilibrium in the body, improving the metabolic rate and giving you more energy. Their high water content, meanwhile, helps to rehydrate the system from within, which further brings a restored and rejuvenated look to the skin – another tick in the box for radish's skin-benefiting powers.

SKIN-FEEDING NUTRIENTS

- Dietary fiber
- Minerals:
  calcium
  copper
  iron
  magnesium
  manganese
  zinc
- Phytochemicals:
  carotenoids
    (alpha- and
    beta-carotene,
    lutein,
    zeaxanthin)

- Vitamins:
  A
  B2 (riboflavin)
  B3 (niacin)
  B6 (pyridoxine)
  B9 (folate)
  C
  E
  K

RADISH SALAD (P. 58)

S ALMON

Good-quality salmon – preferably organic and line-caught – makes all the difference because it tastes so much better, in my opinion. Like other oily fish, it is fabulous for the complexion, too. Regarded as a superfood, salmon contains health-boosting ingredients, in particular omega-3 fatty acids that plump up the skin, boosting production of collagen and elastin and leaving your complexion looking more youthful. It's also a rich source of selenium, which helps to protect and repair sun damage to the skin, as well as helping control irregular pigmentation. A lot of people have pigmentation problems, myself included, so it's great to find something that will help keep unwanted pigmentation at bay or help it fade slightly. Just bear in mind that selenium is not a miracle cure – the best it can do is offer greater protection. Vitamins B5 and B12, also present in salmon, do wonders for hair health and growth, as well as keeping the skin and hair looking glossy and strong, while vitamin D keeps teeth and bones strong and is great for blood-sugar levels, too, which again impacts positively on the skin by reducing sugar spikes that can be so aging for the skin (see p. 16).

SKIN-FEEDING NUTRIENTS

- Fatty acids:
  omega-3
- Minerals:
  iodine
  phosphorus
  selenium
- Protein:
  all nine essential
    amino acids

- Vitamins:
  B5 (pantothenic
    acid)
  B7 (biotin)
  B12 (cobalamin)
  choline
  D

SEAWEED

I love seaweed – it tastes of the sea and feels like a very clean food, as well as being great for the skin. It's full of iodine, a powerful nutrient that supports the thyroid gland. This in turn maintains proper metabolic function, which can impact weight management, mood and energy levels. Worldwide, thyroid problems are common and a lack of iodine is often to blame, though in the West the condition is more likely to be due to issues related to the immune system attacking the thyroid gland. If your thyroid gland is underactive, it can lead to dry skin and premature lines and wrinkles. An underactive thyroid is also associated with fluid retention and puffy skin. Seaweed – including the more popular varieties of nori, kelp and wakame – is also a rich source of other skin-benefiting minerals, such as calcium, magnesium and iron.

SKIN-FEEDING NUTRIENTS

- Dietary fiber
- Minerals:
  calcium
  iodine
  iron
  magnesium
  phosphorus
  potassium

SEAWEED NORI ROLLS (P. 56)

SPINACH

What's the first thing that comes to mind when someone mentions spinach? Popeye, of course! Even in cartoon form it's a symbol of strength and vitality. The fact that it's a dark green vegetable should also signal that it must be good for you, as anything this color is full of vitamins and minerals, including iron. What's useful to remember is that if something's got iron in it, it will move the blood – iron being a key component of hemoglobin – and if it moves the blood, then it will repair the skin. Once you learn about the diversity and density of the nutrients packed into spinach leaves, it's easy to understand how it has earned its reputation as one of the healthiest foods around. Antioxidants like vitamins A and C work to repair skin cells, boost collagen production and keep the complexion looking vibrant and youthful, with improved elasticity. In addition, vitamin K keeps the skin clear, reduces inflammation and enhances blood circulation, while the water content of spinach helps maintain hydration of the skin. The nutrients in spinach also help to keep the eyes healthy and sparkling, and are beneficial for a number of skin conditions, including acne.

SKIN-FEEDING NUTRIENTS

- Dietary fiber
- Minerals:
  iron
  magnesium
- Protein
- Phytochemicals:
  carotenoids
    (beta-carotene)

- Vitamins:
  A
  B9 (folate)
  C
  E
  K

Pearl barley and chocolate porridge

SERVES 2

———

280 CALORIES
PER SERVING
(WITHOUT TOPPINGS)

———

- ½ cup pearl barley
- 1 cup unsweetened almond milk
- 2 tbsp raw cacao (or cocoa) powder, plus extra for sprinkling (optional)
- 1 tsp ground cinnamon

TO SERVE
- Honey (optional)
- Blueberries
- Sliced banana

I love the nutty taste of pearl barley and like to use it in place of other more traditional staples. I make pearl barley risotto (instead of using Arborio rice), for instance, and this pearl barley porridge (instead of using oats). It's such a wholesome and nicely filling way to start the day: made up of complex carbohydrates, rather than rapidly released simple sugars, pearl barley is less likely to cause a blood-sugar spike, too. Here I've served it with chocolate milk for a very yummy breakfast dish. It's a myth that chocolate gives you pimples: raw cacao (used in the luxurious Perfumed Chocolates on p. 132) in particular is rich in nutrients, and contains no sugar. If you find it too bitter, you could add a drizzle of honey, a natural sweetener, to serve.

1. Place the pearl barley and 2½ cups of water in a large saucepan. Bring to a boil, then reduce to a simmer and cook for 20–25 minutes or until the grains are soft and plump. Drain in a sieve to remove any excess water and return to the pan.
2. Pour ¼ cup of the almond milk into a small saucepan and add the cacao (or cocoa) powder and cinnamon. Warm through over low heat, stirring, until the cacao powder has been absorbed.
3. Pour the remaining milk into the pan with the cooked pearl barley and bring to a boil, stirring. Cook until most of the milk has been absorbed, then remove from the heat.
4. Divide the pearl barley porridge between bowls and drizzle over the chocolate milk, adding a drizzle of honey to sweeten, if needed. Top with blueberries or slices of banana and a dusting of cacao (or cocoa) powder, if you wish.

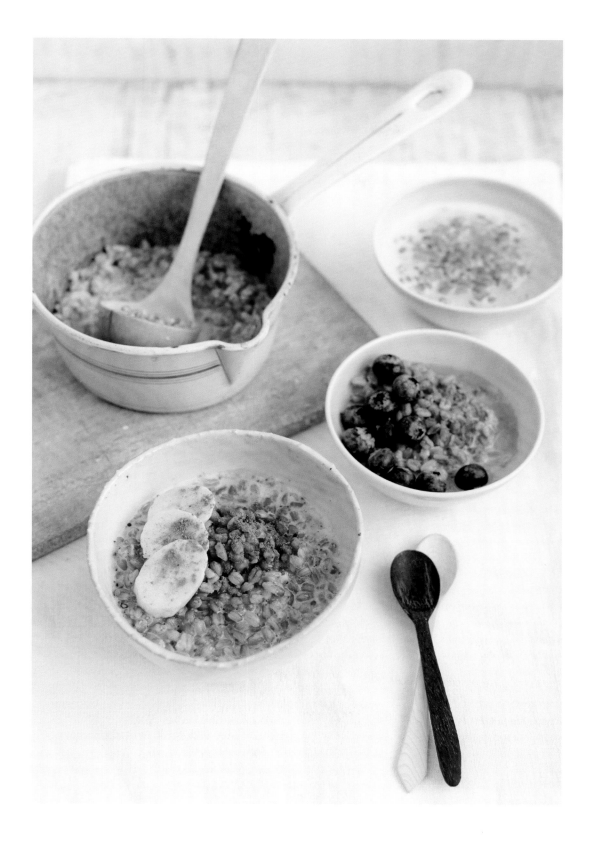

Breakfast wraps

SERVES 1

————

260 CALORIES
PER SERVING

————

- 3 eggs
- 1 tbsp almond milk
- Pinch of sea salt
- Pinch of cayenne pepper
- ½ tsp raw coconut oil
- 1–2 avocados, finely chopped
- Handful of arugula, chopped
- 3 slices of smoked salmon
- 1 tbsp chopped flat-leaf parsley
- Squeeze of lemon juice

This is great for the morning as it gives you the protein you need to start the day. Like salmon, eggs are a good source of selenium and other skin-benefiting nutrients.

1. Whisk the eggs, almond milk, salt and cayenne pepper.
2. Melt the oil in a medium skillet set over medium heat. Pour the egg mixture into the pan, tilting the pan to ensure it covers the base, and cook until golden brown on the bottom before flipping to cook the other side.
3. Transfer to a plate; add the avocado and arugula in a line down the middle. Top with the smoked salmon, parsley and lemon juice, then roll up and cut in half to serve.

Stuffed figs with a fresh basil salad

SERVES 2

————

160 CALORIES
PER SERVING

————

- 4 fresh figs
- 4 slices of Parma ham
- 1 oz goat cheese, halloumi or buffalo mozzarella, chopped
- Large handful of arugula leaves
- Handful of fresh basil

It's funny how life sometimes throws you exactly what you need. While writing this book, I happened to be in a deli in Majorca and a stranger shared this recipe with me. I don't eat much cured meat, but when in Rome – or Spain, as the case may be – I love eating as the locals do. Basil is good to have on hand to sprinkle over pasta or salads; it also makes a great pesto when crushed up with pine nuts and Parmesan (see p. 156). This is delicious, so do give it a go.

1. Preheat the oven to 400°F.
2. Cut a cross in the top of each fig and carefully push your fingers inside to create a cavity. Push a quarter of the chopped goat cheese or other cheese inside each.
3. Wrap each fig in a slice of Parma ham and place it upright on a baking sheet.
4. Place in the oven, reduce the heat to 325°F and cook for 10 minutes. Serve warm on a bed of arugula and fresh basil leaves.

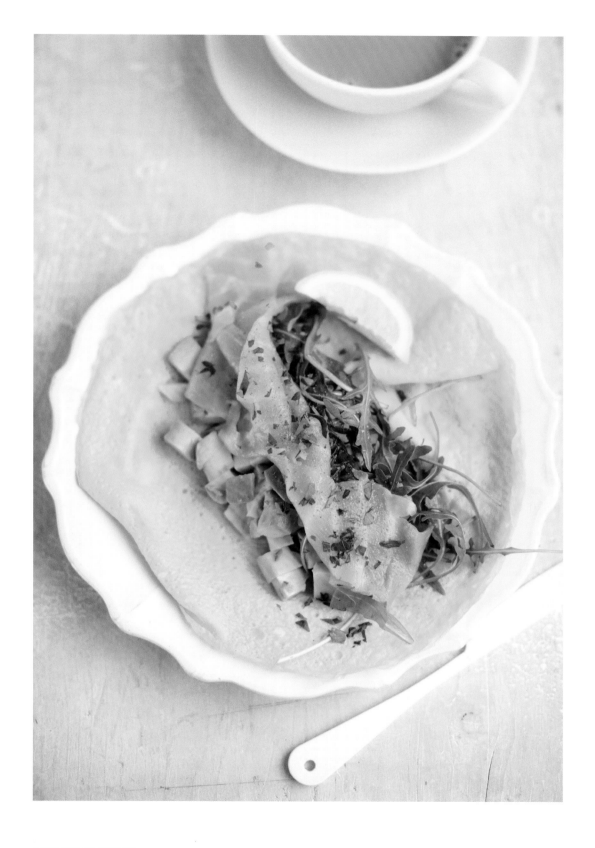

Skin-friendly frittata with salsa verde

SERVES 4

————

480 CALORIES
PER SERVING

————

FOR THE SALSA VERDE
- 2 scallions, finely chopped
- 2 tbsp chopped fresh flat-leaf parsley
- 2 tsp balsamic vinegar
- Juice of ½ lemon
- 1 tsp honey
- 4 tbsp extra-virgin olive oil
- 2 tbsp chopped almonds

FOR THE FRITTATA
- 1 tbsp butter
- 2 leeks, finely sliced
- 2 garlic cloves, finely chopped
- 2 sweet potatoes, peeled and cut into thin strips (see tip)
- ¼ tsp ground cumin
- Leaves from 8 sprigs of thyme
- 8 medium eggs
- Small handful of fresh flat-leaf parsley, finely chopped
- 2 oz Parmesan cheese, grated
- 1 oz artichoke hearts from a jar or can, drained and cut in half
- Sea salt and black pepper

I often make a frittata when I have friends over – it's a wholesome dish that always looks great and so rustic, too. It looks even better served with the bright green parsley salsa verde on top. Onions and leeks contain a type of dietary fiber that acts as a prebiotic within the body, feeding good bacteria and promoting a healthy gut, so vital for the proper absorption of nutrients from food.

1. Preheat the oven to 425°F.
2. Place all the ingredients for the salsa verde in a food processor and blend to the desired consistency.
3. Melt half the butter in a large ovenproof skillet over medium heat. Add the leeks and garlic and cook for 5 minutes until softened, then transfer to a plate and set aside.
4. Melt the remaining butter in the pan, add the sweet potatoes, cumin and thyme and cook over medium-high heat for 5–8 minutes until tender and golden. Remove the pan from the heat.
5. Remove the sweet potatoes from the pan and place on paper towels to absorb some of the moisture.
6. Place the eggs in a bowl with the parsley and Parmesan and whisk together.
7. Transfer the leek mixture and sweet potatoes back into the pan, add the artichoke hearts and mix. Season with salt and pepper and pour in the egg mixture.
8. Place the pan in the oven and bake for 15 minutes or until firm (see tip). Divide between plates and serve with the salsa verde.

TIPS
- Use a mandoline or julienne peeler, if you have one, for slicing the sweet potatoes into thin strips.
- Finish off the frittata under the broiler, if needed, to get it properly crispy on top.
- Reduce the calories by using coconut oil, not butter.

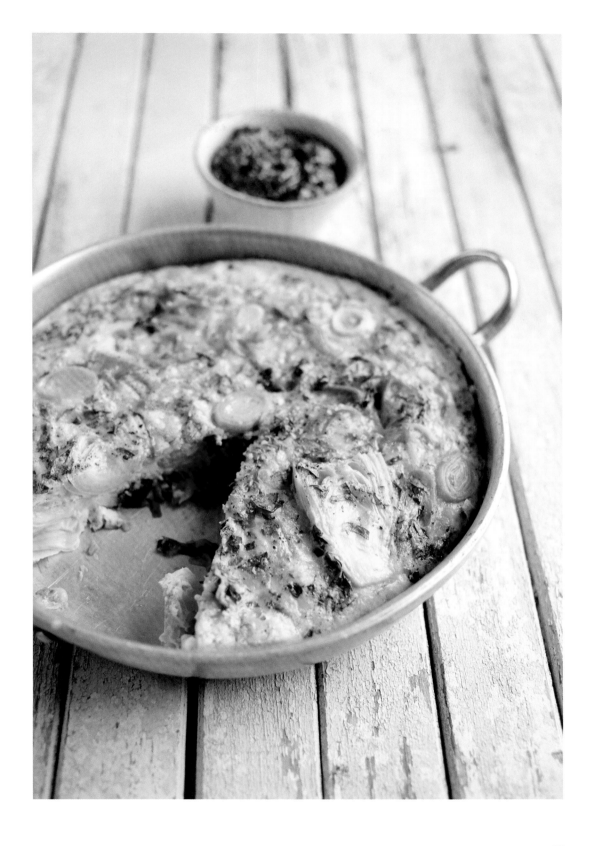

Seaweed
nori rolls

SERVES 4
AS AN APPETIZER

————

358 CALORIES
PER SERVING

————

- ¼ cup sunflower seeds
- ¾ cup raw cashews
- 1 shallot, chopped
- Handful of fresh cilantro, roughly chopped
- Handful of fresh mint, roughly chopped
- 1 tbsp tamari, plus extra for serving
- 2½-inch knob of fresh ginger, peeled and chopped
- 1 tbsp apple cider vinegar
- 4 nori sheets
- 1 carrot, cut into fine batons
- 1 cucumber, cut into fine batons
- 1–4 red cabbage, finely sliced
- Flesh of 1–2 avocado, finely diced
- Handful of alfalfa sprouts

I've personally always adored Japanese food – it's so pure-tasting. Seaweed salads are really quite gorgeous, but if you're not into that rubbery texture then these nori rolls are the simplest way to prepare seaweed. Don't be scared of making your own: this recipe is really straightforward and fun to do with a friend. You just need a bamboo sushi mat to help roll up the sheets of nori. The cashew and sunflower seed "rice" makes a great alternative to the actual grain and, packed with other skin-benefiting ingredients, you know the reward at the end will be a brighter, clearer complexion and a happier metabolism. Tamari is a gluten-free alternative to soy sauce, and hence perfect for those who are gluten intolerant.

1. Place the sunflower seeds and cashews in a food processor with the shallot, herbs and tamari, and process until the mixture has the consistency of cooked rice.
2. Place the ginger in a bowl, add the apple cider vinegar and 1 tablespoon of water and leave to marinate for 10 minutes. Drain.
3. Take a nori sheet and spread one-quarter of the sunflower seed and cashew mixture over it, leaving a ½-inch border around the edges.
4. Place the carrot, cucumber, red cabbage, avocado, alfalfa sprouts and marinated ginger in a line down the middle of the rice mixture. Roll up the nori sheet tightly – using a bamboo sushi mat to help you – and repeat with the three other nori sheets and the remaining vegetables.
5. Cut each roll into five using a sharp knife, and serve with extra tamari.

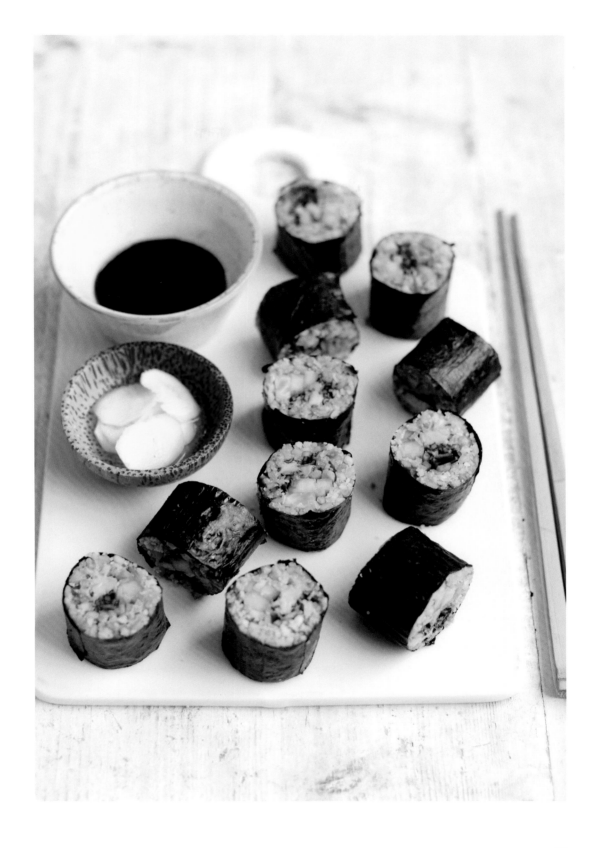

Radish salad

——

85 CALORIES
PER SERVING

——

- 5 radishes
- ½ small cucumber
- Handful of arugula
- Handful of watercress
- Handful of alfalfa sprouts
- Small handful of fresh cilantro, chopped
- Small handful of fresh flat-leaf parsley, chopped
- 1 tbsp flaxseed oil
- Juice of ½ lemon

This salad is brimming with skin-brightening ingredients and tastes as good as it looks. Flaxseed oil is a rich source of omega-3 fatty acids that may help to reduce the symptoms of eczema. Use a mandoline if you have one.

1. Cut the radishes and cucumber into very thin slices and place in a large bowl with the greens and herbs.
2. Just before serving, pour over the flaxseed oil and lemon juice and toss together well.

Speedy leafy greens

SERVES 2

——

80 CALORIES
PER SERVING

——

- 2 handfuls of spinach, roughly chopped
- Handful of curly kale (thick stems removed), roughly chopped
- Handful of chard (stems removed), roughly chopped
- 1 garlic clove, finely chopped
- 1 tbsp extra-virgin olive oil
- ½ tsp crushed red pepper flakes
- Pinch of sea salt
- Squeeze of lemon juice

This is an ultra-healthy and super-fast dish that will give your skin a powerful hit of the best beautifying nutrients there are. (Almost every ingredient has its own section in this book!) I can always put leafy greens into any dish, cooked or uncooked. If I'm being indulgent and I fancy a pizza, for instance, I make sure it's salad-driven by throwing a handful of arugula on top of the cooked pizza to balance out the naughtiness.

1. Place the prepared greens and garlic in a strainer and pour over a kettle of boiling water to blanch.
2. Transfer the greens to a large bowl. Toss together with the olive oil, crushed red pepper flakes and salt. Add a squeeze of lemon juice before serving.

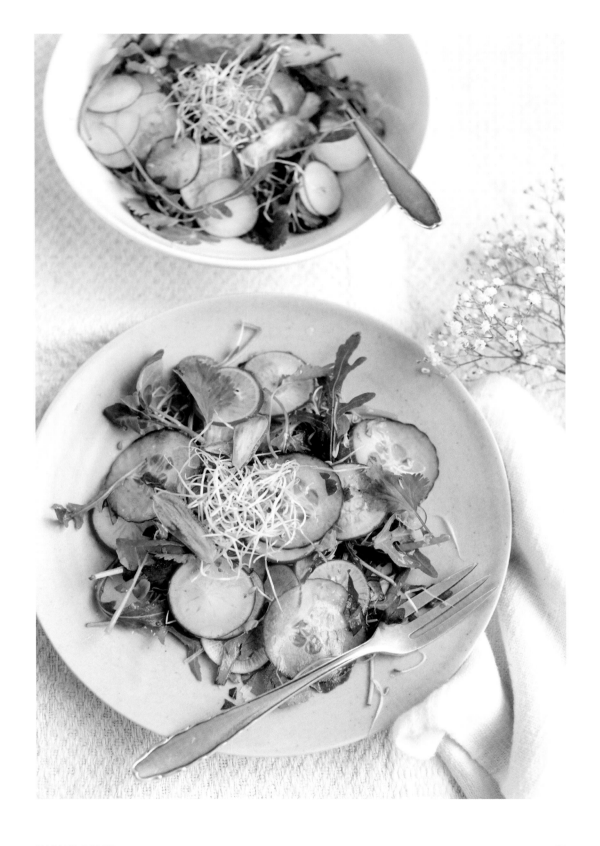

RADISH SALAD

Cilantro and beet salad with avocado and mint

SERVES 2

————

165 CALORIES
PER SERVING

————

- 3 medium-sized cooked beets, thinly sliced or cut into chunks
- ½ medium-sized red onion, thinly sliced
- ¼ cup mâche
- 1 tsp sherry vinegar
- 2 large handfuls of fresh cilantro, torn
- Large handful of fresh mint, torn
- 1 fresh red chile, seeded and finely chopped
- 1–2 tsp sweet chile sauce
- Sea salt and black pepper
- Flesh of 1 small avocado, sliced, to serve

I love fresh cilantro because it reminds me of Thailand and gorgeous Asian food, which always tastes so fresh and clean. I particularly like it in salads, such as this beet and avocado recipe I make all the time. The lively flavor of the fresh herb brings the recipe to life, and I know it's helping to balance my blood sugar as I eat it, while improving the health of my skin, too. Beet, mint and avocado are also all great for the skin, making this dish a real powerhouse for the complexion.

1. In a large bowl, combine the beets, onion, mâche and vinegar.
2. Add the cilantro, mint, chopped fresh chile and sweet chile sauce (to take away the sharpness of the vinegar).
3. Season with a pinch each of salt and pepper and serve with slices of avocado.

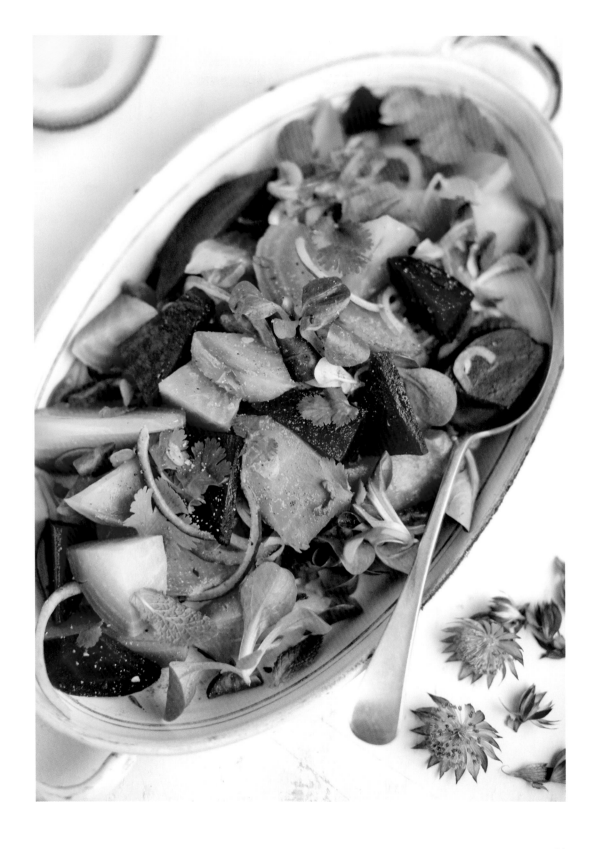

61

Sautéed spinach

SERVES 2
AS A SIDE DISH

——

60 CALORIES
PER SERVING

——

- 2 tsp raw coconut oil
- 1 garlic clove, finely chopped
- 4 handfuls of spinach
- Pinch of crushed red pepper flakes
- Pinch of sea salt

You can eat spinach in so many ways: younger leaves in a salad, and bigger leaves in a curry, added to quinoa or rice, or juiced. It is a rich source of beta-carotene, an antioxidant nutrient essential for healthy skin that is absorbed more efficiently in the presence of fats – hence the coconut oil.

1. In a large pan, melt the oil. Add the garlic and spinach and cook over medium heat for 2 minutes or until the spinach has wilted.
2. Chop up the spinach in the pan, season with the crushed red pepper flakes and sea salt and serve immediately.

Herby arugula salad

SERVES 2
AS A SIDE DISH

——

150 CALORIES
PER SERVING

——

- 4 handfuls of arugula
- Handful of baby spinach
- Small handful of fresh parsley
- Small handful of fresh cilantro
- Small handful of fresh mint
- 1 tbsp sunflower seeds
- ¾ oz Parmesan cheese, shaved
- 1 tbsp extra-virgin olive oil
- 1 tsp balsamic vinegar

When it comes to arugula, I prefer keeping it simple. I always include it as a side when ordering pizza – not just to make me feel less guilty, but because the leaves are high in fiber, helping my body to digest the fat and carbs. Arugula is also super low in calories. When not enjoying the peppery leaves on their own, I mix them with skin-benefiting spinach and herbs for a fresh-tasting salad that's full of aromatic flavor – a real tonic for the metabolism and for your skin.

1. Throw all the green leaves and herbs into a bowl and toss to combine.
2. To serve, sprinkle with the sunflower seeds and Parmesan shavings and dress with the olive oil and balsamic vinegar.

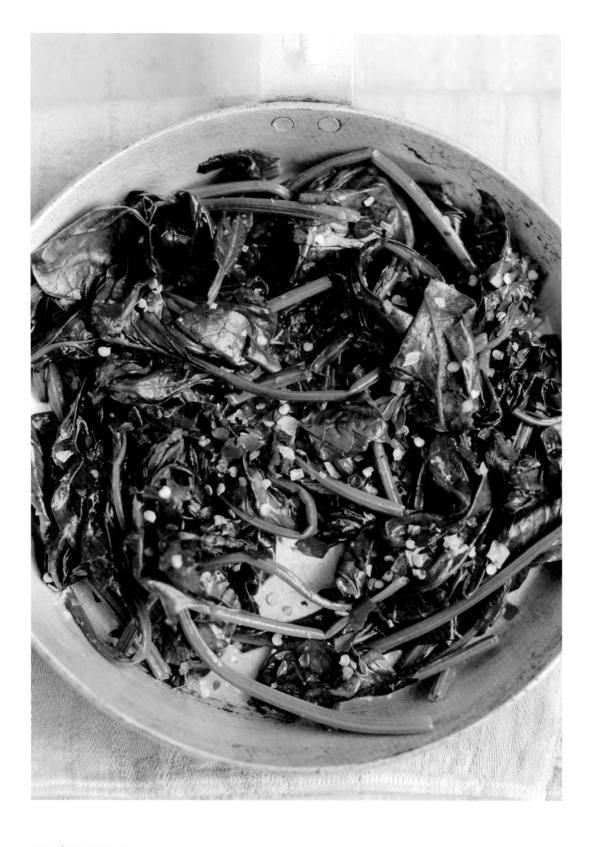

SAUTÉED SPINACH

Baked eggplant

SERVES 2

———

433 CALORIES
PER SERVING

———

- 2 eggplant, sliced
  in half lengthwise
- 2 tbsp olive oil
- 1 cup quinoa
- 1 vegetable stock cube
- 2 shallots, chopped
- 2 handfuls of spinach
- 2 garlic cloves, chopped
- ½ oz Parmesan cheese

The meatiness of eggplant feels substantial and is extremely good for nourishing the skin as well. You can prepare and cook the filling the night before.

1. Preheat the oven to 400°F.
2. Place the eggplant, cut side up, on a baking sheet. Drizzle with oil and bake for 20 minutes or until tender.
3. Meanwhile, place the quinoa in a pan and add the stock cube and 1½ cups of water. Bring to a boil, reduce the heat and simmer for 20 minutes. Cook covered for the last 5 minutes to make the quinoa sticky.
4. When the eggplant are done, scoop out the insides, leaving the skins on the baking sheet. Transfer the flesh to a food processor and add the shallots.
5. Put the spinach and garlic in a sieve and pour boiling water over to blanch. Add to the processor and whizz until smooth. Place in a bowl and stir in the quinoa.
6. Grate the Parmesan into the quinoa mix before spooning back into the eggplant skins. Bake for another 5 minutes or serve immediately.

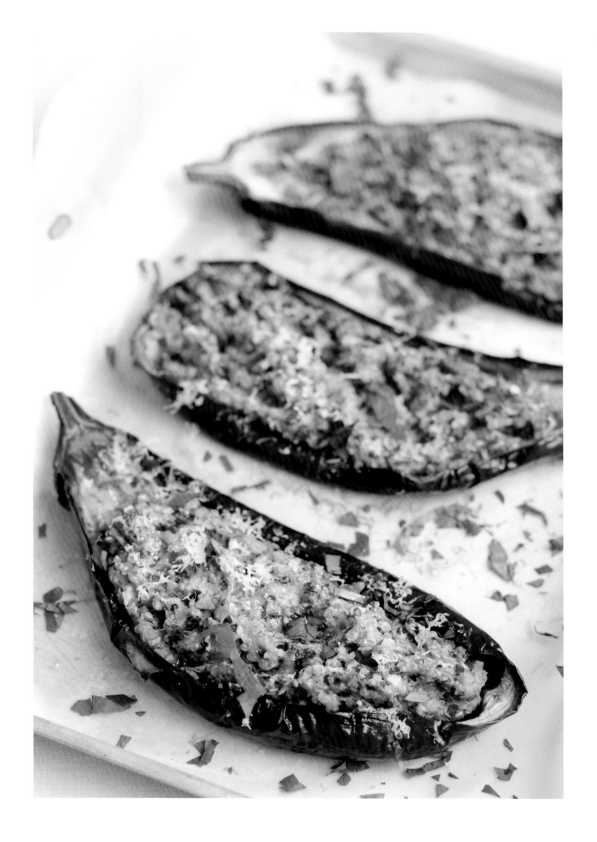

Almond chocolate milkshake

SERVES 1

————

150 CALORIES
PER SERVING

————

- Handful of ground almonds
- ¾ cup unsweetened almond milk
- 1 tbsp raw cacao (or cocoa) powder, plus extra for sprinkling (optional)
- 1 tsp honey

I love mixing raw cacao powder with almond milk to make this chocolate drink. It contains nothing that will aggravate the skin – just a touch of honey as a natural alternative to sugar – but is full of nutrients and tastes completely delicious, too.

1. Place everything in a blender and whizz until smooth. Sprinkle additional cacao powder on top before serving, if desired.

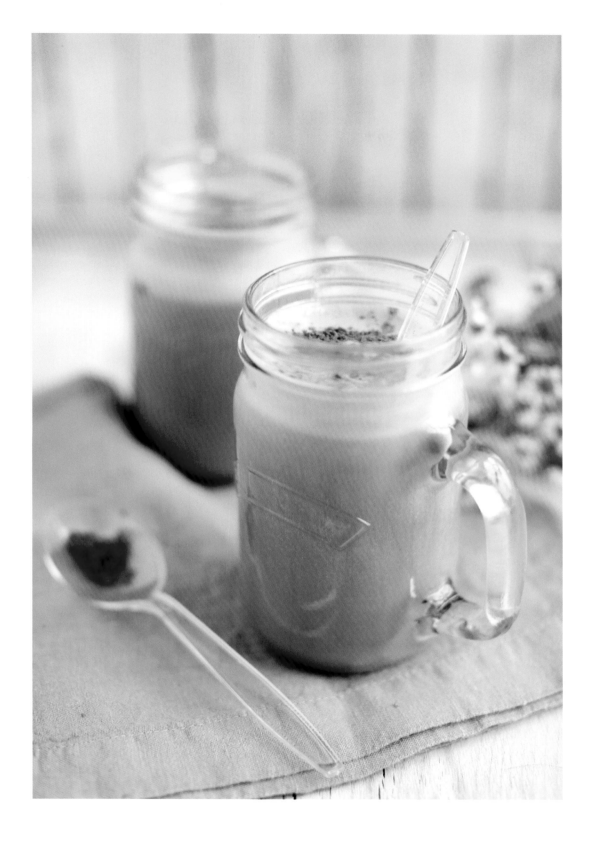

Quinoa with pesto chicken

SERVES 2

————

640 CALORIES
PER SERVING

————

- ¾ cup quinoa
- 1 tsp extra-virgin olive oil
- 2 skinless and boneless
  chicken breasts,
  cut into 1-inch pieces
- 2 handfuls of arugula
- 2 oz buffalo mozzarella,
  torn into pieces
- ½ oz Parmesan cheese
- 2 tsp flaxseeds
- Handful of alfalfa sprouts
- 1 tsp flaxseed oil, to serve

TO SERVE
- 3 tbsp of Pine Nut Pesto
  (p. 156) or store-bought
  fresh pesto

This was a recipe that I came up with on a day when I really needed comfort food but I didn't want to succumb to temptation and order my takeout favorite – pizza. This is a healthy, filling meal, rather than a pure carbs and fat option, because that was what I really needed. Containing skin-benefiting chicken and alfalfa (see pp. 141 and 84), in addition to the quinoa, it's rich in protein and in dietary fiber, helping to retain a feeling of fullness and control blood-sugar levels, and thereby avoid energy slumps and sugar cravings.

1. Place the quinoa in a medium saucepan and pour in 1½ cups of water. Bring to a boil, then reduce the heat and simmer for 15–20 minutes or until it is tender and all the water has been absorbed. Remove from the heat and set aside, covered with a lid to keep warm.
2. Meanwhile, heat the oil in a large, deep-sided saucepan and add the chicken. Cook over medium heat for 12–15 minutes, stirring frequently, until golden in color and cooked through. Add the pesto to the pan and stir in to coat the chicken pieces.
3. Add the pesto chicken to the cooked quinoa, followed by the arugula and mozzarella, and stir to combine. Grate over the Parmesan and scatter over the flaxseeds and alfalfa sprouts before drizzling with the flaxseed oil to serve.

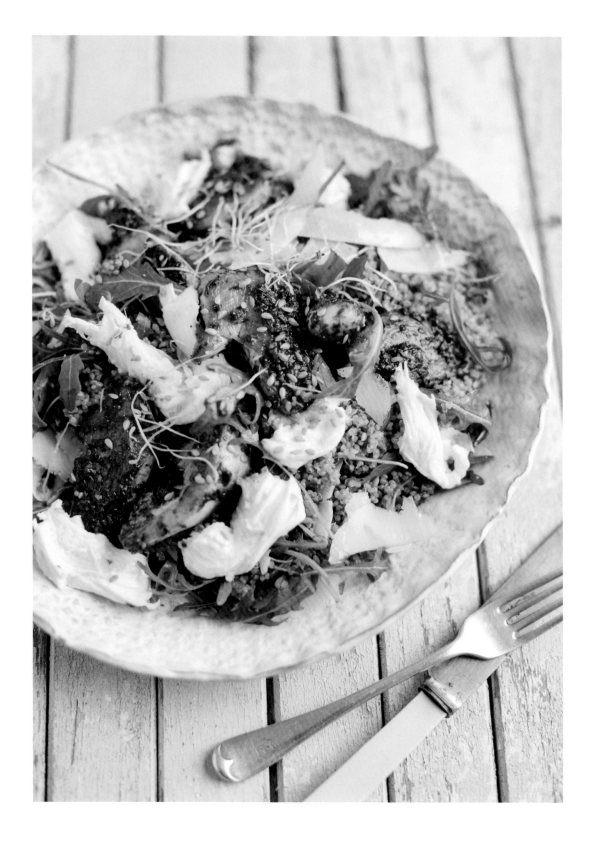

Salmon with asparagus and fennel

SERVES 2

————

460 CALORIES
PER SERVING

————

- 2 skinless salmon fillets
- 1 tbsp grated fresh ginger
- 1 tsp Chinese five-
  spice powder
- ½ tsp ground turmeric
- 2 tbsp raw coconut oil
- 1 fennel bulb, finely sliced
- 5 asparagus spears, chopped
  into 1-inch lengths
- 1 tbsp tamari sauce
- Grated zest of 1 lemon
- ¼ cup coconut milk

TO SERVE
- 2 tsp flaxseed oil
- Small handful of fresh
  basil, roughly torn

I love how asparagus spears are pretty much ready as they are. Very little is needed in the way of preparation or cooking – the simpler the better, in fact. Grilled with a little olive oil and scattered with a sprinkling of Parmesan, they're good to go. They also make great barbecue food for an appetizer before the meat is ready. If not eating asparagus on its own, I love pairing it with salmon – another miracle food for skin. Like asparagus, fennel – also included in this dish – is a great diuretic and has many other skin-healthy properties, too.

1. Add the salmon to a bowl and toss with the ginger and spices.
2. Melt the coconut oil in a large, deep-sided skillet and add the salmon. Cook on each side over medium heat for 5 minutes or until just cooked through, then remove the salmon and set aside on a plate, covered in foil.
3. Place the fennel and asparagus in the pan and pour in ½ cup of water. Add the tamari and lemon zest, then bring to a simmer, cover the pan with a lid and cook gently for 10 minutes.
4. Remove the lid and pour in the coconut milk. Bring back up to a simmer and continue to cook for 2 minutes.
5. Divide the cooked vegetables between bowls and place a salmon fillet on top of each. Drizzle with the flaxseed oil and scatter with the basil to serve.

    ASPARAGUS (P. 34)

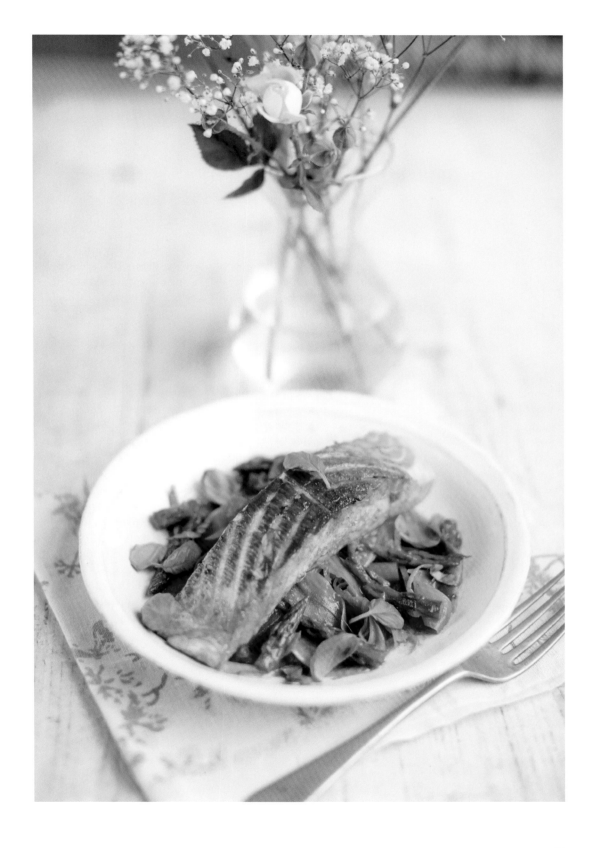

Beet
and quinoa
burgers

MAKES 4 BURGERS

———

260 CALORIES
PER BURGER

———

- ¼ cup quinoa
- 5 tbsp ground flaxseed
- 6 tbsp warm water
- 1 eggplant, chopped
- 3 medium-sized cooked beets, grated
- 2 garlic cloves, finely chopped
- ½ cup gluten-free rolled oats
- Oil, for cooking
- Sea salt and black pepper

TO SERVE
- 4 slices of buffalo mozzarella
- 4 large spinach or lettuce leaves

If you're like me, you sometimes want something filling but not too naughty. The earthy, meaty texture of beets is perfect. Oats are great for the skin, too. These do take a little time to make but are worth it.

1. Place the quinoa in a medium pan and pour in ¾ cup water. Bring to a boil, then simmer for 15–20 minutes or until tender.
2. Add 2 tablespoons of the flaxseed to a small bowl with the warm water, stir together and set aside.
3. Steam the eggplant for 5 minutes until tender enough to pierce with a fork, then transfer to a food processor and whizz until smooth. Place in a bowl and set aside.
4. Now blitz the beet. Add the garlic, oats and final 3 tablespoons of flaxseed. Pulse to combine, then transfer to a large bowl. Add the soaked flaxseed and eggplant and season. Mix together to form a dough.
5. Shape into four burgers, then place on a parchment paper-lined baking sheet. Chill in the fridge for at least an hour.
6. Pour oil into a large skillet over medium heat (or work in batches if you don't have a skillet large enough to fit all four burgers comfortably). When hot, add the burgers and sear on each side for 3–4 minutes.
7. Top with a slice of mozzarella and wrap in a leaf to serve.

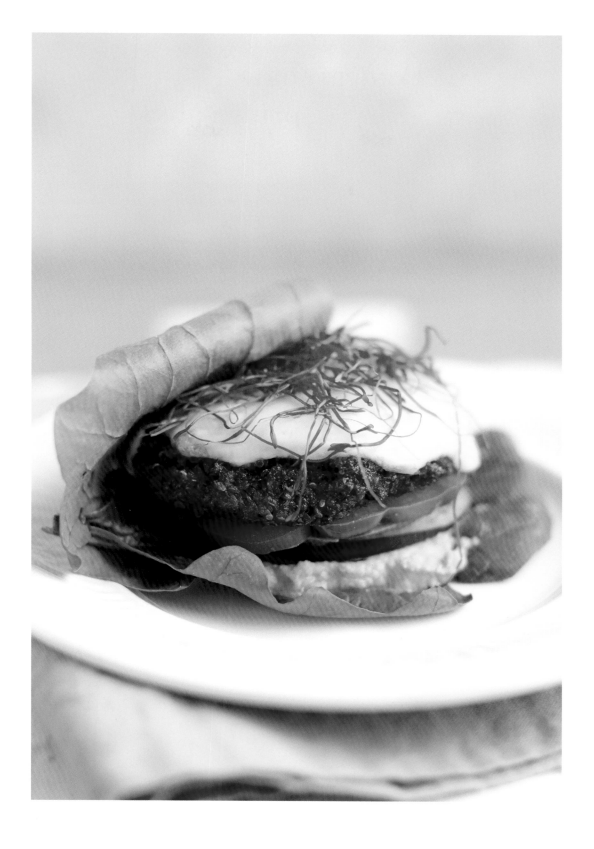

Pomegranate
spring salad

SERVES 2

———

400 CALORIES
PER SERVING

———

- 1 cup quinoa
- 1 garlic clove,
  finely chopped
- Handful of
  pomegranate seeds
- Handful of spinach,
  roughly chopped
- Handful of fresh mint,
  chopped
- Handful of fresh
  cilantro, chopped
- Handful of fresh
  parsley, chopped
- 1 tbsp flaxseed oil
- 1 tbsp ground flaxseed
- Sea salt

I love to sprinkle pomegranate seeds into salads and grain dishes. They add a touch of sweetness and, being bright in color, they always make the dish look more vibrant.

1. Place the quinoa in a medium saucepan with 1½ cups of water, the garlic and a pinch of salt. Bring to a boil, then reduce the heat and simmer for 15–20 minutes or until tender and all the water has been absorbed.
2. Allow the quinoa to cool and then place in a bowl. Add the pomegranate, spinach and herbs and mix together.
3. Drizzle over the flaxseed oil and sprinkle with ground flaxseed to serve.

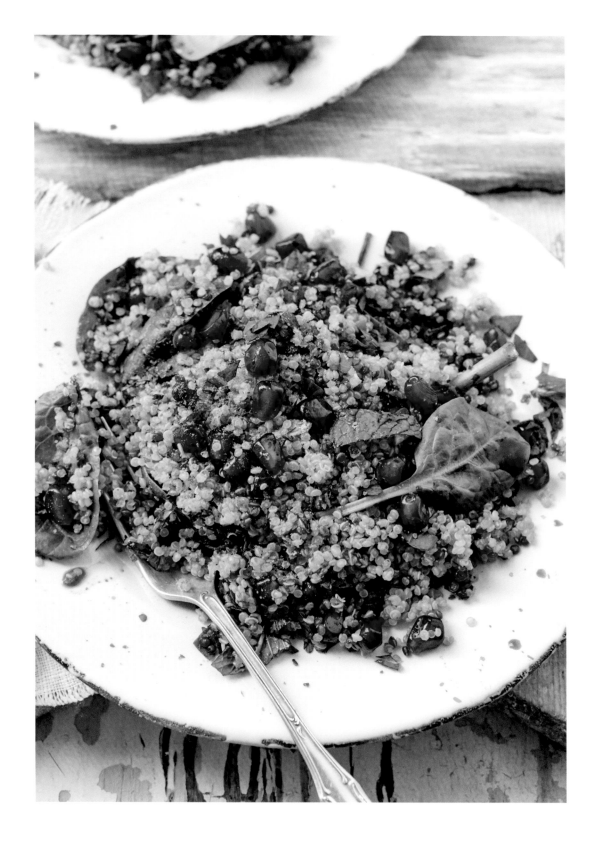

Savory
popcorn

SERVES 2

———

250 CALORIES
PER SERVING

———

- 1 tbsp olive oil
- ½ cup popcorn kernels
- ½ tbsp vegetable
  bouillon powder
- 1 tsp crushed red pepper
  flakes

This is a great recipe because you can make it at home, from the best-quality popcorn, and take it with you to the movies in a zip-top bag – I've yet to find a movie theater that sells organic popcorn. The only downside is that, like all popcorn, it's utterly moreish – I can't stop helping myself to great handfuls of it, so that when the lights come up, it's all over me! It is also really quick to make!

1. Place the oil in a large saucepan over medium heat. Add the popcorn kernels and cover the pan with a well-fitting lid. Shake the pan to coat the corn in the oil and leave for about 4 minutes until all the kernels have popped.
2. Once the popping sound slows down, remove the pan from the heat and leave for a few minutes to cool slightly.
3. Pour the popcorn into a large resealable freezer bag and add the bouillon powder and crushed red pepper flakes. Shake to ensure the popcorn is well coated and then transfer to a large bowl to serve.

GLUTEN-FREE "POP" CRUMBS
A fun, gluten-free alternative to bread crumbs in a recipe is crushed popcorn. People get a real kick out of it when you tell them what your chicken or fish is coated in!

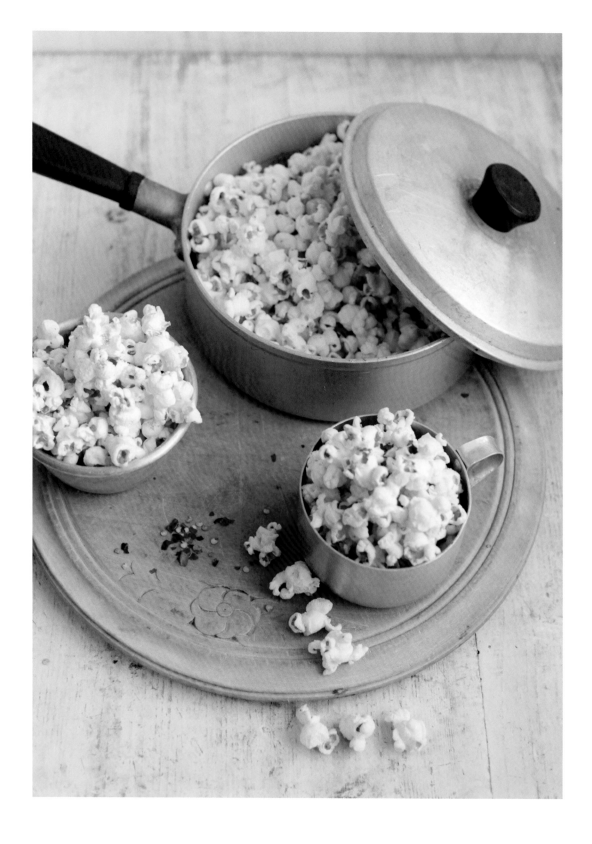

77 of 276

77

Blueberry milkshake

SERVES 1

———

178 CALORIES
PER SERVING

———

- Handful of blueberries
- ¾ cup unsweetened almond milk
- 1 date, pitted
- 1 tbsp ground chia seeds
- Sprig of mint, to decorate

For a great start to my morning, I like to throw a handful of blueberries in a blender with some almond milk – giving me a boost in energy and a hit of anti-aging nutrients. This couldn't be any quicker.

1. Place all the ingredients except for the mint in a blender and whizz until smooth.
2. Serve topped with a sprig of mint.

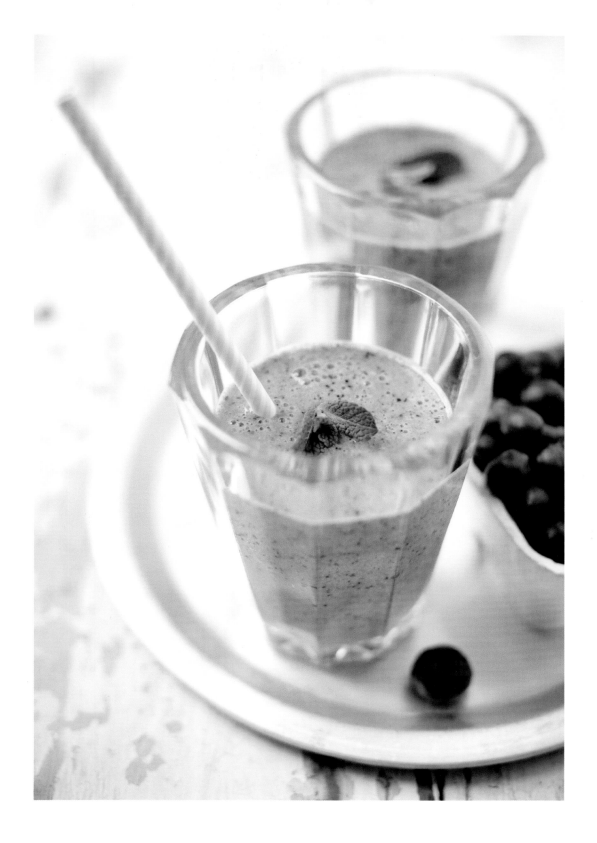

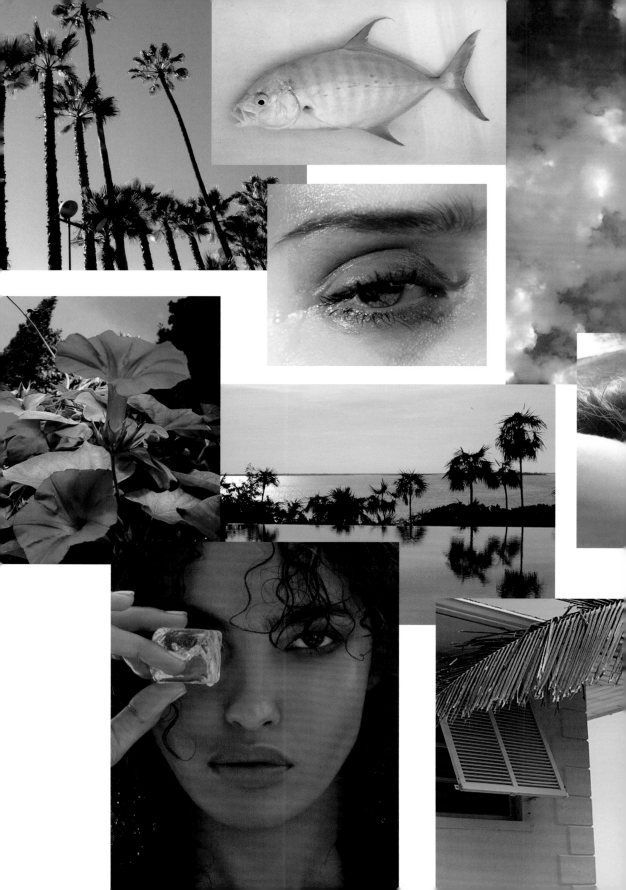

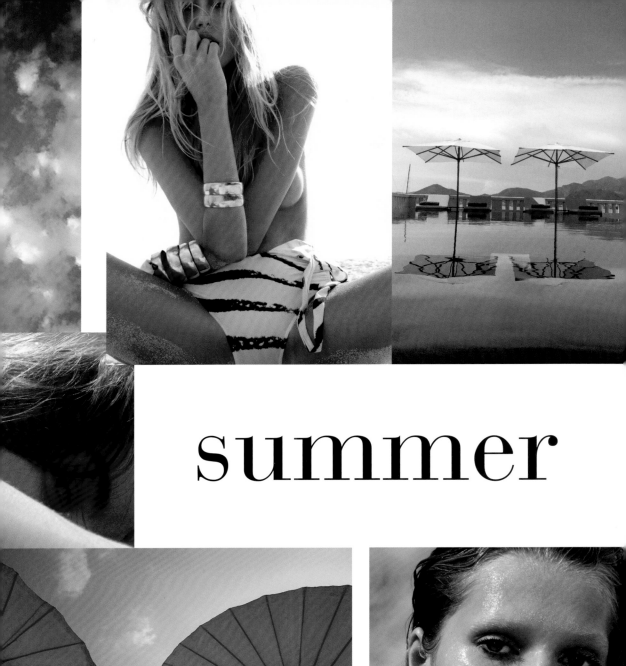

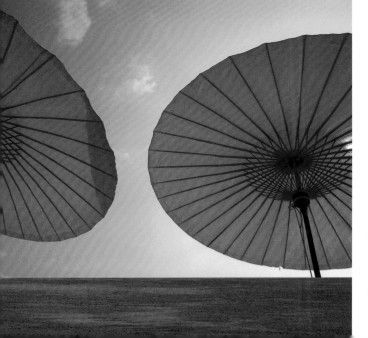

summer

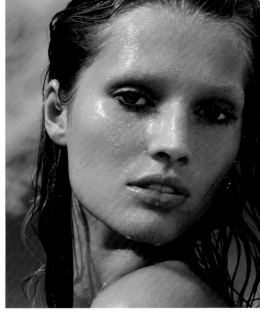

Eat your water

I look forward to the summer – longer days and more time outdoors. The sun changes your mood, putting a smile on everyone's face. During the summer months it's important to consume more water. It's not just about drinking: I believe that we can "eat our water" with a diet of fresh fruit and vegetables. I take advantage of having less appetite and opt for salads and vegetable juices, not stodgy grains and hard-to-digest meats.

Many factors can take a toll on the skin during the summer: greater UV exposure, higher temperatures and dryness from air-conditioning can result in sun damage, dehydration, oiliness from extra sebum secretion and breakouts.

Select foods rich in selenium, zinc and vitamins C and E, nature's protectors against free-radical-producing UV rays. Lycopene, for instance – a phytochemical present in some red fruits and vegetables – is believed to increase protection against UV by boosting levels of pro-collagen. Of course, it's important to use a broad-spectrum sunscreen, too, especially for UVA protection. The damage caused by overexposure to these long-wave rays of ultraviolet light, such as premature *aging* or an increased risk of skin cancer, may not appear for years. UVB short-wave rays are the type of ultraviolet light that causes *burning*. But as we all know, it's easy to get caught up in other activities (sitting on a terrace, chatting with friends or eating outside); often it's not until you take a shower that you realize you're sunburned. Rather than getting unattractive pigmentation on your face, which is really tough to get rid of, it's better to be safe than sorry. So apply a good sunscreen, regularly topped up, and eat generous quantities of rehydrating fruit and veg!

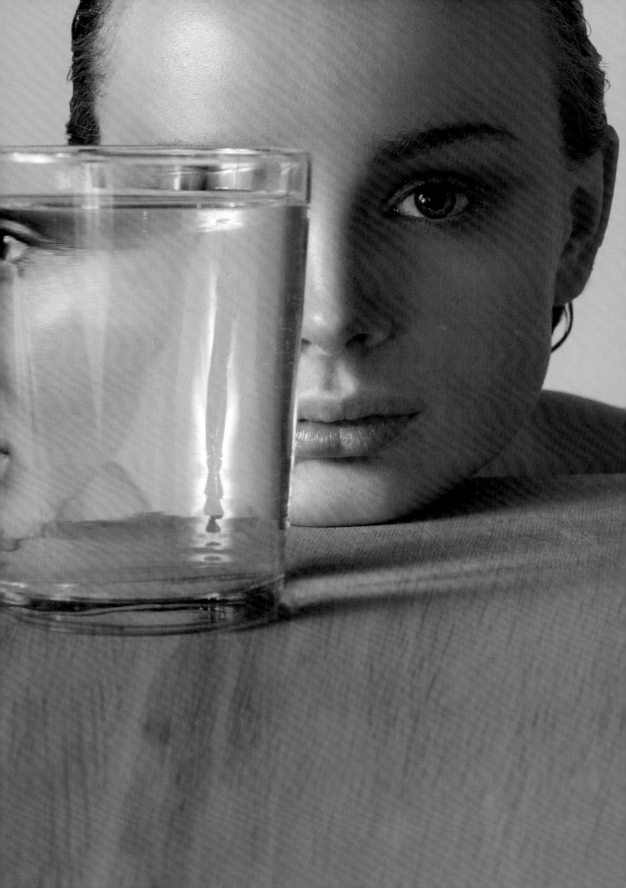

ALFALFA

THE MINI SUPERHERO

Alfalfa is a clover-like plant that's been grown around the world for centuries as a forage crop. I'm not suggesting you eat the fully grown plant, but the sprouting seeds – increasingly available in supermarkets – are definitely worth including in your diet. You can use them just as you would mustard and watercress; there's no cooking involved and the benefits are major. I personally try to include them in as many fresh recipes as I can – especially in juices to add a more green/earthy flavor. They don't have a particularly distinctive taste, so they are really easy to mix in with any kind of salad. Once you learn how brimming with powerful plant actives and skin-benefiting nutrients these little guys are, you'll understand their appeal. Packed to the rafters with amino acids, vitamins, a whole array of different minerals and phytochemicals, there's not much the mighty alfalfa can't do. Known to detoxify and alkalize the blood, alfalfa acts as a diuretic, helping relieve fluid retention, and supports healthy blood-sugar levels, as well as being anti-inflammatory and antifungal in its effect. Alfalfa is often used as a base in vitamin and other "food state" supplements due to its rich nutrient and enzyme content, which is easily absorbed by the body in this form.

SKIN-FEEDING NUTRIENTS

- Dietary fiber
- Minerals:
  calcium
  copper
  iron
  magnesium
  phosphorus
  potassium
  silica
  sulfur
- Protein:
  all nine essential
    amino acids

- Vitamins:
  A
  B1 (thiamine)
  B2 (riboflavin)
  B3 (niacin)
  B9 (folate)
  choline
  C
  E
  K

ALFALFA CHICKEN PITA (P. 116)

AVOCADO

THE INNER MOISTURIZER

I'm probably preaching to the converted when I recommend eating more avocados – they've become super popular in recent years, but it wasn't always so. Back in the not too distant past, they were considered a dietary no-no thanks to their high fat content, which was previously thought to be a fast track to gaining weight. But of course, newer research has confirmed that fats – that is, good fats like those found in avocados – are not only beneficial for us, but are essential for many bodily functions, and can even help us to lose weight, not gain it (as long as you don't eat loads). But it's not only our waistline that benefits from the humble avocado – it is extremely effective for the skin, too. Containing monounsaturated fatty acids that work together to keep the skin moist and healthy and to protect skin against UV damage, avocados soothe any symptoms of sensitivity and inflammation at the same time. Rich in antioxidants, they help to protect against cell damage of the skin and the ravages of free radicals; they also promote skin elasticity. All in all, avocado makes a great addition to your diet – you could describe it as an internal moisturizer. Most of the models I work with would wholeheartedly agree. You can use avocados externally, too – they are known to work very well when applied topically to the skin as a moisturizing face mask.

SKIN-FEEDING NUTRIENTS

- Dietary fiber
- Fatty acids:
  monounsaturated
    (oleic acid)
  omega-3
- Minerals:
  copper
  magnesium
  potassium
- Phytochemicals:
  carotenoids
    (alpha- and
    beta-carotene,
    beta-cryptoxanthin,
    lutein, zeaxanthin)
- Vitamins:
  B2 (riboflavin)
  B6 (pyridoxine)
  B7 (biotin)
  C
  E
  K

GUACAMOLE (P. 104)

B ANANA

THE HANGOVER CURE

If you ask just about anyone why bananas are healthy, most people will say it's because they're full of potassium – and they're right, of course, but there are many other nutritional reasons to make bananas a part of your diet. Potassium is an important mineral for regulating nerve function, supporting the cardiovascular system and lowering blood pressure. But bananas are also rich in other essential nutrients: they contain high levels of vitamin C and B6, for instance, which support the elasticity of the skin as well as restore its natural radiance. Meanwhile, the vitamin A content helps to repair dull and damaged skin, and restores natural hydration for a more supple look. It's the banana's ability to flush the body, owing to the fiber it contains, and its high natural sugar content that make it particularly helpful for a hangover; when the liver is struggling to get the body back on form and you're craving something sweet after drinking too much alcohol, a banana is just the thing to help restore the body's equilibrium. The tryptophan a banana contains is necessary for producing serotonin, the "feel-good" hormone, so you should feel better, too!

SKIN-FEEDING NUTRIENTS

- Dietary fiber
- Minerals:
  manganese
  potassium
- Protein:
  amino acids
    (tryptophan)

- Vitamins:
  A
  B6 (pyridoxine)
  B12 (cobalamin)
  C

FROZEN BANANA ICE POPS (P. 130)

BLACK-EYED PEA

Black-eyed peas may make me think of a certain hip-hop band rather than the original foodstuff – a pale-colored bean with a distinctive black "eye" or spot in the middle. I was introduced to them (the beans, that is) through friends whose parents were from the West Indies, as they're used a lot in Caribbean cooking, such as the recipe I've included here. They tend to be labeled a health food, and for good reason as they are full of nutrients, making them an excellent addition to any skin-focused diet. High in soluble fiber and low in calories, they help to regulate blood-sugar levels, which not only makes us feel better and on more of an even keel, but it stops the skin from erupting into the angry breakouts that can follow a blood-sugar spike. They're known for their ability to help delay signs of aging due to the high protein content, which helps with growth and repair of tissues in the body, making them the perfect food to eat if you're vegetarian or don't consume much meat. They're a rich source of vitamins and minerals, too – you know you're getting a good hit of what your skin and body needs every time you eat them, plus they leave you feeling nicely full and less likely to reach for a sweet treat when your blood sugar drops.

SKIN-FEEDING NUTRIENTS

- Dietary fiber
- Minerals:
  calcium
  copper
  iron
  magnesium
  manganese
  phosphorus
  potassium
  selenium
  zinc
- Protein
- Vitamins:
  A
  B1 (thiamine)
  B2 (riboflavin)
  B3 (niacin)
  B9 (folate)
  C
  K

BROWN STEW CHICKEN WITH
BLACK-EYED PEA RICE (P. 122)

Cucumber

Is there anything as refreshing in summer as a cucumber? With a water content of 95 percent, this is the very best foodstuff to consume if you want to rehydrate through eating, in addition to drinking water. Often overlooked as being of little nutritional significance, cucumbers are packed with a host of skin-feeding vitamins and nutrients, too. Known for their ability to reduce inflammation and eliminate toxins, cucumbers can help deal with digestive problems such as acid reflux and constipation, meaning that they help to flush the system like an internal cleanser, creating a less acidic environment in the gut. They are packed with antioxidants – powerful actives that work to combat the free radicals that cause aging – while cucumber skin contains one of the richest sources of silica, a mineral that activates enzymes involved in the production of collagen (maintains skin structure and elasticity). There's a good reason for the age-old practice of placing slices of cucumber over the eyes during downtime – it's particularly effective in reducing eye puffiness, the vitamin C and caffeic acid helping to relieve fluid retention for an instant tightening and refreshing effect. A natural soother for sunburn when applied to the skin, cucumber also works to treat open pores when applied topically, too.

SKIN-FEEDING NUTRIENTS

- Minerals:
  magnesium
  manganese
  phosphorous
  potassium
  silica
- Phytochemicals:
  caffeic acid
  carotenoids
    (alpha- and beta-
    carotene, lutein,
    zeaxanthin)

- Vitamins:
  A
  B5 (pantothenic acid)
  C
  K

CUCUMBER AND MANGO SALSA (P. 126)

DARK CHOCOLATE

Is there anyone on earth who doesn't like chocolate? If there is, I haven't met them. So it will undoubtedly bring much joy to many to hear that chocolate is good for the skin. Of course that doesn't mean cheap, sugary chocolate, but the high-quality, low-sugar or unsweetened, dark variety with at least 85 percent cocoa solids (the higher the percentage, the better it is for you), which is packed full of antioxidants that can be a powerful anti-aging treatment for the skin. Rich in nutrients, high-quality dark chocolate can protect the skin from damaging UV rays, while also working to firm and repair the complexion. The anti-inflammatory properties help to reduce inflammation in the body, making it an excellent resource in the fight against skin conditions like rosacea and eczema. You might have heard that chocolate prompts the body to release the hormone dopamine, which is responsible for feelings of satisfaction and happiness – much like the feeling after sex, when the hormone is also released! It's been suggested that on top of this dopamine release, chocolate can increase the production of mood-enhancing neurotransmitters, so there are legitimate reasons why we instinctively reach for the chocolate when feeling low. Reducing stress hormones – like cortisol – means the skin is less at the mercy of the collagen breakdown that is linked to this process: happy mind equals happy skin. It's important to note that it needs to be low in sugar, high in cacao and consumed in moderation. So if you eat homemade ones like mine, with only natural sweeteners, you'll find them so rich that one or two will be enough.

SKIN-FEEDING NUTRIENTS

- Dietary fiber
- Fatty acids: monounsaturated (oleic acid)
- Minerals:
  calcium
  copper
  iron
  magnesium
  potassium
  sulfur
  zinc
- Phytochemicals:
  flavonoids
  polyphenols
- Vitamins:
  A
  B1 (thiamine)
  B2 (riboflavin)
  B3 (niacin)
  B5 (pantothenic acid)

PERFUMED CHOCOLATES (P. 132)

FENNEL

THE WONDER BULB

They don't call this the "flat stomach" vegetable for nothing. If you suffer from bloating, try eating fennel – it's a great diuretic for the body. Fennel has been used for centuries – particularly by women – for many reasons, quite apart from its distinctive anise-like flavor. I'd been ignoring it for ages because I didn't really know what to do with it, until I discovered that it adds an amazing creaminess to soup, as you'll see from the recipe I've included on page 113. It's also delicious cooked on its own – drizzled in olive oil and roasted – or you can use the seeds to add flavor to dishes. As well as helping with fluid retention, fennel has been used throughout history as a libido-booster, a hormone balancer and a cure-all for skin conditions. An excellent source of vitamins, especially vitamin C, the plant is known for its anti-aging properties, along with its antiseptic and diuretic qualities, making it the perfect addition to a weight-loss regimen. Loaded with essential minerals each with their own special function in keeping the skin clear, glowing and blemish-free, fennel can also help to keep the face from looking puffy. The seeds, nutritious in their own right, can be used as a breath freshener – in fact there are some Indian restaurants that offer them after a meal for this purpose, which I love.

SKIN-FEEDING NUTRIENTS

- Dietary fiber
- Minerals:
  calcium
  copper
  iron
  magnesium
  potassium
  zinc
- Vitamins:
  A
  B6 (pyridoxine)
  B9 (folate)
  C

FENNEL AND CELERY SOUP (P. 113)

FIG

THE INNER EXFOLIATOR

Juicy sun-ripened figs remind me so much of summers spent in Majorca, where the fruit grows everywhere. I hated figs as a kid; my only experience of them was in dried form in the processed filling of fig rolls – a favorite of my dad's – or something dried that you ate to make you go to the toilet. Of course, as a child I didn't care about the importance of "being regular." Oh, how things have changed since then! These days you're able to buy fresh figs much more easily, especially in southern climes. I have a few glamorous friends – mentioning no names – with places abroad that have quite amazing gardens with fig trees growing in them. You don't need to be glamorous to have fig trees, of course, and you don't even need fig trees – just a good supplier. Figs are full of fiber, so I don't feel guilty about eating the sweet fruit because it will flush through me in a day, and anything that moves through the body really quickly, allowing it to absorb other nutrients more efficiently, is always good. Anything that flushes through the system also helps to detoxify the skin, making figs excellent for treating skin conditions like psoriasis or acne. In addition to the roughage they contain, the fresh fruits provide natural sweetness, making them a brilliant way to sweeten dishes as an alternative to refined sugar.

SKIN-FEEDING NUTRIENTS

- Dietary fiber
- Minerals:
  calcium
  magnesium
  phosphorus
  potassium

- Vitamins:
  A
  B1 (thiamine)
  B2 (riboflavin)
  B3 (niacin)
  C

K IWI

THE SKIN BRIGHTENER

I love how kiwis are so portable: a very handy little fruit – one for the handbag! You eat them as you would a boiled egg – just cut the top off and all you need is a teaspoon. Definitely something to bear in mind as, super rich in vitamin C, they are one of the major fruits for your skin, with an even higher content than an orange. A powerful antioxidant known for its ability to protect and brighten skin, vitamin C is needed for the growth and repair of tissues through collagen production. Our bodies can't produce vitamin C, and aren't able to store it either, so regular consumption of foods containing this vitamin, such as the kiwi, is essential. Vitamin C is also great for general wound healing and helps with sun damage and unwanted pigmentation, too – another reason to make it part of a good summer diet. Meanwhile, the minerals they contain are another element in the array of nutrients required for maintaining healthy skin. The kiwi fruit can be mashed up and applied to the skin directly. It's important to wait until the kiwi is ripe, however, because its properties become more powerful, with greater benefit to the skin. So don't forget: a kiwi a day keeps the wrinkles away!

SKIN-FEEDING NUTRIENTS

- Dietary fiber
- Minerals:
  calcium
  copper
  magnesium
  potassium

- Vitamins:
  C
  K

KIWI PANCAKES (P. 102)

LIME

THE NATURAL ASTRINGENT

Like all citrus fruit, limes are an excellent addition to any dish, thanks to their unique zesty flavor. And while the metabolism-boosting benefits of drinking water with lemon juice first thing are well known, it's easy to overlook limes, which have the same nutritional qualities as lemons. In cooking both lemons and limes have the ability to keep things light and refreshing – particularly in the warmer months. Citrus fruit are excellent for the complexion – they're rich in powerful antioxidants such as vitamin C and citric acid, which work to keep the skin clear of congestion and impart a natural glow. Thanks to their natural antibiotic properties, limes can help prevent acne by keeping the bacteria that causes breakouts at bay. Their natural astringency helps keep the skin looking taut and firm by causing a minute, temporary tightening of the muscles, which also works to tighten pores and reduce oil secretion. We tend to assume citrus fruit have an acidic effect on the body when ingested, but they're actually alkaline, meaning they aren't acid-forming but quite the opposite, making them a great addition if you are following an alkaline diet. To me limes quite simply feel "clean" – like they're doing you good from the inside out. Able to help fight free radicals owing to their high levels of vitamin C, they help contribute to overall health and a brighter, more youthful-looking complexion.

SKIN-FEEDING NUTRIENTS

• Dietary fiber
• Phytochemicals:
  citric acid
  flavonoids
• Vitamins:
  C

MINT

THE STOMACH CALMATIVE

Looking through these recipes, you may have noticed how much I enjoy adding mint to my dishes. I love the fresh taste and how it works like a palate cleanser to cut through other flavors, all the while promoting efficient digestion and reducing inflammation. The distinctive herb has a long history of use in cooking: there's even a Greek myth dedicated to it, while the Romans were responsible for creating the mint sauce we still eat today. Known especially for its digestive-calming properties, mint is what I always go for when I have an upset stomach. A sprig of fresh mint in some hot water tastes great and works quickly to settle the digestion – it even helps to treat motion sickness when traveling by plane or boat. A real Florence Nightingale of the herbs. The phytochemicals carvacrol, thymol and menthol also enhance the calming effect of mint in tackling flatulence – just the thing if you're feeling a bit bloated after a meal. Growing a pot of mint on a windowsill or in the garden is a great way to ensure it's always on hand to mix into salads, sprinkle onto sorbet or infuse to make into a tea, as it is a very vigorous herb. Given half a chance, it will grow like wildfire. Get more mint in your diet – your stomach will thank you and your skin will, too!

SKIN-FEEDING NUTRIENTS

- Dietary fiber
- Minerals:
  calcium
  iron
  manganese
  potassium
- Phytochemicals:
  carvacrol
  menthol
  thymol
- Vitamins:
  A
  C
  B1 (thiamine)
  B2 (riboflavin)
  B3 (niacin)
  B9 (folate)

FRESH MINT PETITS POIS (P. 112)

PARSLEY

THE WONDER HERB

Along with its lively flavor, parsley is so jam-packed with wonderful nutrients that it's worth recasting the frilly green herb as a key ingredient in its own right – like the Italians do in their salsa verde or the Lebanese in their tabbouleh. Crammed with vitamin C – the skin brightener – parsley works from within to nourish the skin and fight signs of aging. It also helps with maintenance and repair of the skin, promoting cell turnover and collagen production for improved overall elasticity. Eating plenty of parsley helps to balance excess sebum secretion in oily skin, due to its vitamin A content, keeping the pores clear and helping to prevent acne outbreaks. The zinc in parsley performs a similar function, controlling inflammation, reducing redness and preventing breakouts – particularly helpful in the treatment of rosacea. Other nutrients also help to lighten shadows under the eyes and reduce puffiness for a more sparkly, bright-eyed look. It's a win-win ingredient: great-tasting and great for the skin and body, too.

SKIN-FEEDING NUTRIENTS

- Dietary fiber
- Minerals:
  calcium
  copper
  iron
  magnesium
  manganese
  potassium
  phosphorus
  zinc
- Phytochemicals:
  carotenoids
    (beta-carotene)

- Vitamin:
  A
  B1 (thiamine)
  B2 (riboflavin)
  B3 (niacin)
  B5 (pantothenic acid)
  B6 (pyridoxine)
  B9 (folate)
  C
  E
  K

WHITE FISH WITH PARSLEY BUTTER (P. 120)

THE COLLAGEN-BOOSTING BERRY

STRAWBERRY

When my sister and I were kids growing up in Essex, we used to go strawberry-picking. While picking we would, of course, try to eat as many strawberries as we could. Afterward my mum would sprinkle them (those we hadn't already eaten!) with sugar and perhaps a drop of single cream, or she would use them to make strawberry jam. Not only are strawberries a summertime institution at events like Wimbledon and completely delicious in the bargain, they're also known to enhance the complexion, thanks to their many skin-boosting nutrients and anti-inflammatory properties. They're a rich source of vitamin C, a known radiance-restoring vitamin that also fights the free radicals that age skin and destroy collagen. Full of dietary fiber, they aid digestion and the detoxification process, too, further helping skin to stay clear and pimple-free. The folate in strawberries helps speed up cell regeneration and the production of new cells; it also prevents collagen destruction and addresses UV damage. Something to think about when you next have a bowl of these gorgeous summer berries!

SKIN-FEEDING NUTRIENTS

- Dietary fiber
- Phytochemicals: flavonoids (ellagic acid)
- Vitamins:
  B9 (folate)
  C
  K

STRAWBERRY SALAD WITH BALSAMIC VINEGAR AND FRESH MINT (P. 128)

T OMATO

I've spent quite a bit of time in Italy, where I've been introduced to tomatoes in a whole range of shapes and colors and learned how to mix them in a wonderful collaboration of different flavors. When you get your hands on beautifully ripe tomatoes in the summer, it's best to keep the dish simple, in my view, to focus on their glorious flavor. But tomatoes also have so many wonderful nutrients that help the skin, too, which is another reason to enjoy them. A rich source of vitamins A and K and the B-complex vitamins, along with the minerals potassium, magnesium, iron and phosphorus, tomatoes help with so much – both beauty and overall health. Aiding the body's natural detoxification process, which is hugely helpful for the health of the gut and the skin. Lycopene, the red pigment in tomatoes, has an antioxidant effect that helps the skin's natural UV defense, and is even thought to help shield the body from certain cancers. The vitamin A in tomatoes is also helpful if you have acne because it reduces the production of sebum, which makes the skin oily.

SKIN-FEEDING NUTRIENTS

- Dietary fiber
- Minerals:
  iron
  magnesium
  phosphorus
  potassium
- Phytochemicals:
  carotenoids
    (lycopene)
- Vitamins:
  A
  B1 (thiamine)
  B3 (niacin)
  B5 (pantothenic acid)
  B6 (pyridoxine)
  C
  K

WATERMELON

Few fruits are so closely associated with a particular season as watermelon is with the summer. The spectacularly colored fruit is a real all-arounder: it tastes fresh and clean, it's easy to use in sweet or savory dishes (or on its own), it's full of water *and* contains skin-feeding nutrients. When I drink a glass of freshly juiced watermelon, it feels as though it's rushing through my system, rehydrating and replenishing as it goes. As I've mentioned previously (see p. 82), when it comes to the skin it's really important to "eat" your water, so foods like watermelon (made up of 93 percent water) are the perfect thing. It is great for rehydration and is particularly useful in the summer when the body and skin are prone to losing moisture. Containing vitamins A and C, the watermelon gives the skin exactly what it needs for a radiant and youthful glow, thanks to its collagen-boosting properties. The lycopene in this fruit protects the skin from UV damage, acting like an internal sunscreen that, combined with topical sunscreens, helps keep the skin from burning. Interestingly, watermelon is a source of iron, increasing red blood cell production, which in turn boosts circulation, promoting healthy skin, hair and nails. Watermelon seeds are little nutritional powerhouses in their own right: they contain beneficial fatty acids and antioxidants that keep the skin hydrated and can help acne sufferers. So don't spit them out – crunch them up with the knowledge they're also doing your skin some good.

SKIN-FEEDING NUTRIENTS

- Minerals: magnesium
- Phytochemicals: carotenoids (lycopene)

- Vitamins:
  A
  B1 (thiamine)
  B6 (pyridoxine)
  C

WATERMELON SALAD (P. 110)

WHITE TEA

When I first lived in the States, friends would offer me either white or black tea, and I wouldn't know which to choose. Where I'd come from, a cup of tea was just a cup of tea – that calming old British faithful. The difference between white and black tea, it seems, is that black tea has been allowed to oxidize so it has a richer flavor, while white tea is a younger leaf that tastes more naturally sweet. White tea provides a boost to energy, because the leaves haven't had a chance to grow, so it is rich in polyphenols, the most abundant type of antioxidant in the diet. It has less caffeine than coffee, so it is always going to be good. Loaded with antioxidants – even more than green tea – white tea can also help fight free radicals, protect the heart and lower cholesterol and it strengthens the immune system, too. White tea is also believed to enhance weight loss and reduce the symptoms of gum disease. Certain types of white tea are known for their anti-aging skin benefits – some people even call them "beauty teas" for their known complexion-boosting nutrients. What more can I say about tea other than it being quintessentially British? It's the traditional restorative: "Have a cup of tea – it's going to be all right." And most of the time it is.

SKIN-FEEDING NUTRIENTS

- Phytochemicals:
polyphenols (catechins)

WILD RICE

THE MINERAL-RICH GRASS

Calling this ingredient "wild rice" is a bit misleading, as it's not really rice, but a type of edible grass – a wonderful grain, in fact. You might notice that it's less available to buy and more expensive than standard rice, which is because it is trickier to grow (in the shallow waters of a lake) and harvesting and processing (to remove the hard, inedible husk) are more labor intensive. So it's worth picking up a package whenever you see one, as it's quite a special food, and full of nutritional value. A rich source of protein, iron and calcium, as well as high in dietary fiber, wild rice is ideal for those looking for good plant-based alternatives to meat, as it's full of nutrients without the inflammation that comes with eating lots of meat. It can be difficult to track down – most major supermarkets don't have it, so when you find a source make sure you stock up. Packed with zinc – which is important for the immune system as well as the health of the hair, nails and skin – it helps to control the production of sebum, making wild rice a great choice for anyone looking to treat acne through diet.

SKIN-FEEDING NUTRIENTS

- Dietary fiber
- Minerals:
  iron
  magnesium
  phosphorus
  potassium
  zinc
- Protein
- Vitamins:
  A
  B1 (thiamine)
  B2 (riboflavin)
  B3 (niacin)
  B9 (folate)

WILD RICE SALAD (P. 106)

THE REHYDRATOR

ZUCCHINI

Zucchini are a brilliant summer addition to any skin-feeding diet. I love cooking with them, too – shredded into a salad, chopped into thick sections for a hearty goulash, or roasted and drizzled in oil. Did you know that a zucchini, also known as "summer squash," is technically a fruit? The great thing about eating fruit/veg from the squash family in summer is that they're so high in water (over 90 percent water content) and low in calories that you can eat as much as you like with zero guilt. A ¾ cup serving of zucchini delivers 37 percent of the required daily intake of vitamin C and over a gram of dietary fiber – at only 20 calories. The "eat your water" principle (see p. 26) is particularly applicable to zucchini because of the high water content, helping to rehydrate your body and skin in the summer months. They are packed with other nutrients, too – in its skin especially (never peel a zucchini for this reason). Diabetics and those who suffer from blood-sugar peaks and troughs should eat more, as the zucchini has properties that are all useful in regulating blood sugar and in breaking down sugars already in the body – and for reducing inflammation, too. The skin's favorite vitamins – A, B complex and C – help fight free radicals and inflammation for that healthy glow, while protecting against the signs of aging from within.

SKIN-FEEDING NUTRIENTS

- Dietary fiber
- Minerals:
  calcium
  copper
  magnesium
  manganese
  phosphorus
  potassium
- Phytochemicals:
  carotenoids
    (beta-carotene,
    lutein,
    zeaxanthin)
- Vitamins:
  A
  B6 (pyridoxine)
  B9 (folate)
  C
  K

ZUCCHINI AND BROWN RICE SPAGHETTI (P. 118)

Kiwi pancakes

MAKES 4 PANCAKES

————

183 CALORIES
PER PANCAKE

————

- 2 tbsp coconut flour
- 4 tbsp buckwheat flour
- 1 date, pitted
- 2 eggs
- ½ cup unsweetened almond milk
- 1 tsp raw coconut oil

TO SERVE
- 2 kiwi, peeled and sliced
- Blackberries
- Natural Greek yogurt
- 4 sprigs of mint

I enjoy eating kiwi just as it is – scooping out the delicious tangy-sweet flesh with a teaspoon. On the weekend, when I have more time, I'll make these pancakes and add some berries and yogurt for a gorgeous relaxed breakfast; the natural sweetness is all that's needed to bring it to life – no sugar necessary. Combining blackberries and kiwi delivers a mega dose of free radical–busting antioxidants, topped off with probiotic-rich Greek yogurt for a feast for the skin!

1. Place the flours, date and eggs in a food processor and pour in the milk and ½ cup of water. Blend all the ingredients together until smooth and transfer to a jar.
2. Melt the coconut oil in a medium nonstick skillet. Pour or ladle enough pancake batter into the pan to cover the bottom of it in a thin, even layer.
3. Cook the pancake over medium heat for 3–4 minutes or until golden brown on the bottom, then carefully flip over using a spatula and cook the other side for another 2–3 minutes. Slip on to a plate and continue making pancakes until the batter is used up.
4. Serve the finished pancakes with slices of kiwi, a sprinkling of blackberries and a spoonful of Greek yogurt. Garnish each one with some mint.

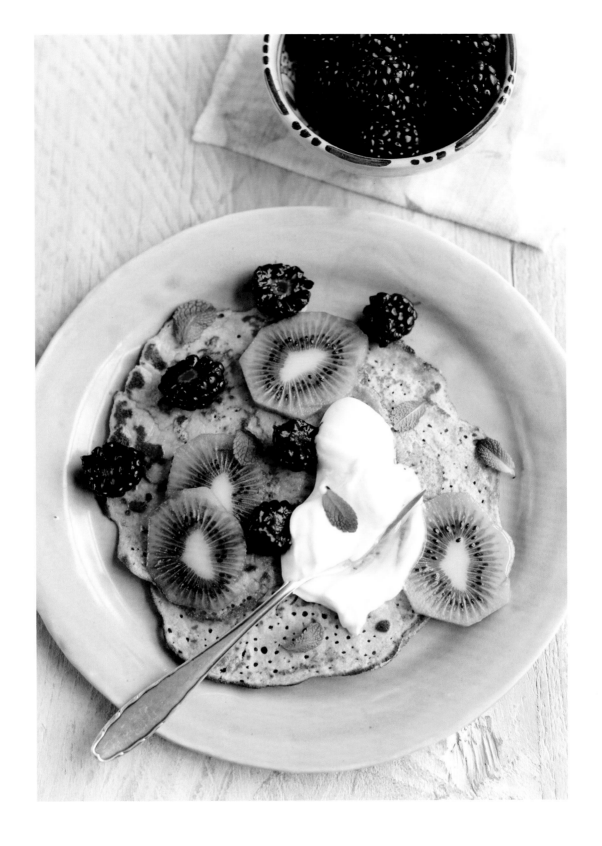

Guacamole

SERVES 4
AS A SIDE DISH

––––

222 CALORIES
PER SERVING

––––

- Flesh of 2 large avocados
- Juice of ½ lemon
- 1–2 fresh red chiles, seeded and finely chopped
- Pinch of paprika
- Small handful of fresh cilantro, finely chopped
- 1 garlic clove, finely chopped
- 1 shallot, finely chopped
- 1 tbsp extra-virgin olive oil
- Sea salt and black pepper

TO SERVE
- Assorted crudités, such as endive, cucumber, asparagus, carrots, and radishes

I always have an avocado at home after a long flight, simply sliced in half with a bit of smoked salmon. The fashion industry is wise to my love of avocados, too, making sure they are always available on shoots among the catering options – I'm clearly a notorious avo addict!

1. Place all the ingredients in a medium bowl and mash together with a fork until the desired consistency is reached, seasoning with salt and pepper to taste.
2. Serve with assorted crudités on the side.

DAIRY-FREE ALTERNATIVE TO BUTTER
Try avocado spread on bread or crackers. I mash it on toast with cayenne pepper and pink Himalayan salt.

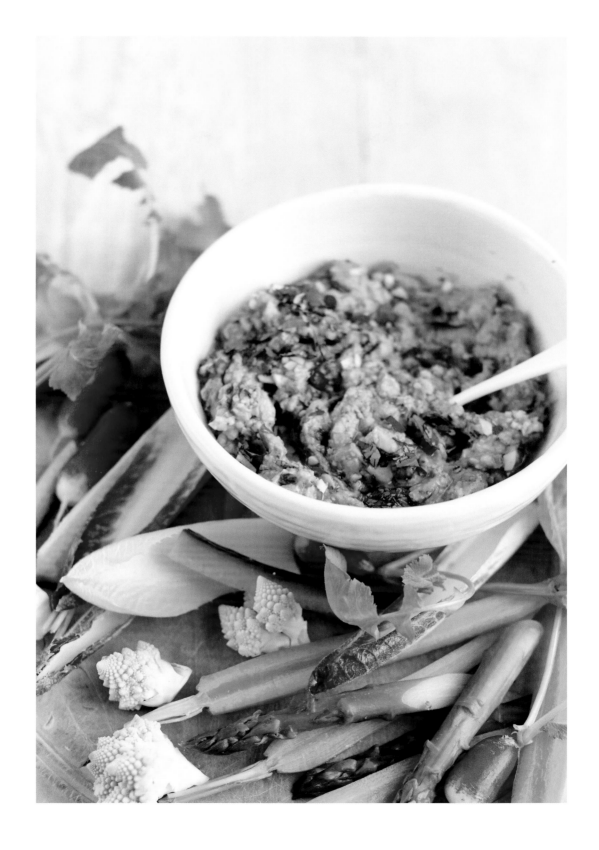

Wild rice salad

---

440 CALORIES
PER SERVING

- ½ cup wild rice
  and ½ cup brown rice
  (or 1 cup mixed brown
  and wild rice)
- 1 tbsp pistachios
- Juice of ½ lemon
- Handful of fresh mint,
  roughly chopped
- Handful of arugula,
  roughly chopped
- ½ garlic clove,
  finely chopped
- 2 handfuls of dried
  fruit such as raisins,
  goji berries, dried
  cranberries or chopped
  dried apricots
- 1 tbsp extra-virgin
  olive oil
- Sea salt and black pepper

This is one of my friend Dom's signature dishes and it is a real winner. The gorgeous nutty texture of wild rice works so perfectly – a great addition to a summer barbecue.

1. Boil each rice in lightly salted water following the package instructions. Drain and rinse under cold water.
2. Meanwhile, toast the pistachios in a small skillet over medium heat for 2–3 minutes, tossing frequently so that they don't burn. Remove and lightly crush.
3. Place the rice in a serving bowl, add the lemon juice, mint, arugula, garlic and dried fruit, and combine well.
4. Drizzle over the oil, then season and sprinkle the toasted nuts over the top to serve.

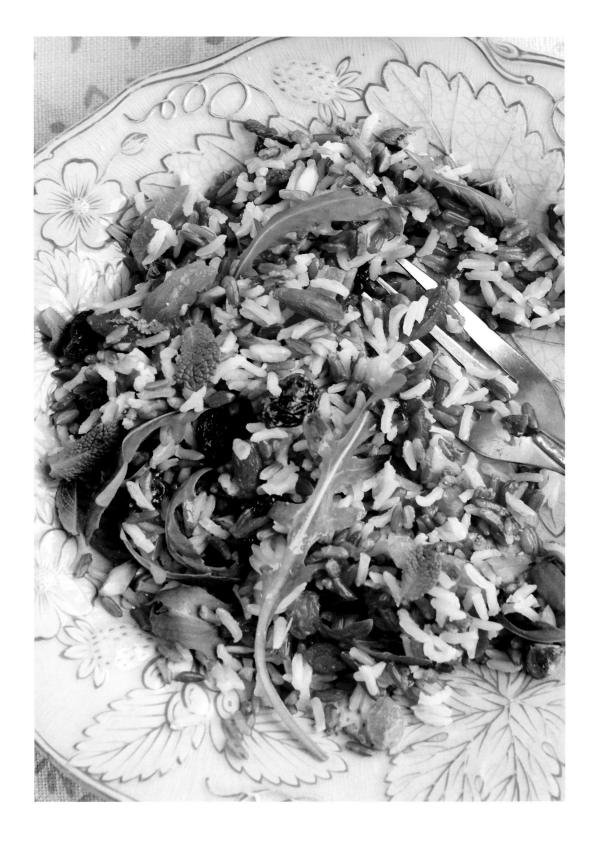

Fresh herb and tomato bites

SERVES 4
AS AN APPETIZER

————

400 CALORIES
PER SERVING

————

- 7 oz ripe tomatoes (preferably in different colors and sizes)
- 2 shallots, finely chopped
- 2—3 garlic cloves, finely chopped
- Handful of fresh basil, chopped
- 2 tsp fresh lime juice
- A good pinch of salt
- 1—2 tbsp extra-virgin olive oil
- 10—12 gluten-free crackers, to serve

This snack is so simple, but that's the beauty of it. There are no tricks, just gorgeous ripe tomatoes doing their thing – not to mention skin-benefiting garlic, basil and lime – tasting delicious and making you look beautiful!

1. Chop up any large tomatoes and quarter cherry tomatoes, then combine in a bowl with the shallots, garlic, basil, lime juice, salt and olive oil. Cover with plastic wrap and set aside for 1 hour for the flavors to meld.
2. Top the crackers with the tomato mixture and serve.

TIPS
- If you are in a hurry, don't worry about waiting for the flavors to meld; just serve immediately.
- These bites are great for a party, as they are simple and quick to prepare.

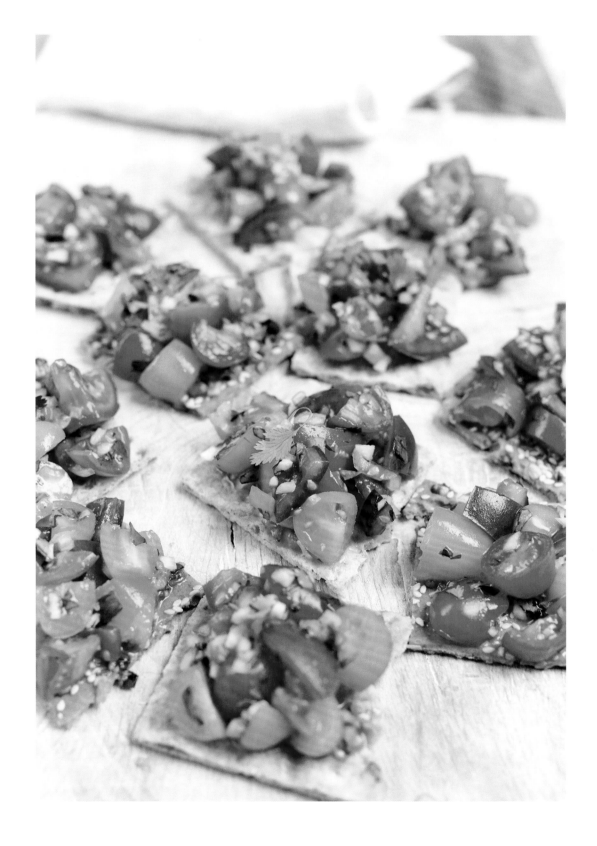

Watermelon salad

SERVES 2

————

382 CALORIES
PER SERVING

————

- 1 lb watermelon flesh, cut into chunks
- Leaves from 1 bunch of mint, larger leaves torn
- Handful of watercress
- 1 tbsp extra-virgin olive oil
- 2 tsp flaxseeds

I love this salad – sustaining and full of what your skin needs after a day in the sun. Watermelon is a great help in restoring the radiance to your skin. Try to eat organic watermelon whenever possible and keep the seeds in because they are really high in iron, which will boost your blood circulation and rejuvenate your skin. This salad is super quick to make.

1. Toss the watermelon, mint and watercress in a bowl.
2. Serve drizzled with oil and sprinkled with flaxseeds.

SUNBURN TREATMENT
Watermelon can be used direct on the skin to soothe sunburn – a great alternative to aloe vera (see p. 256).

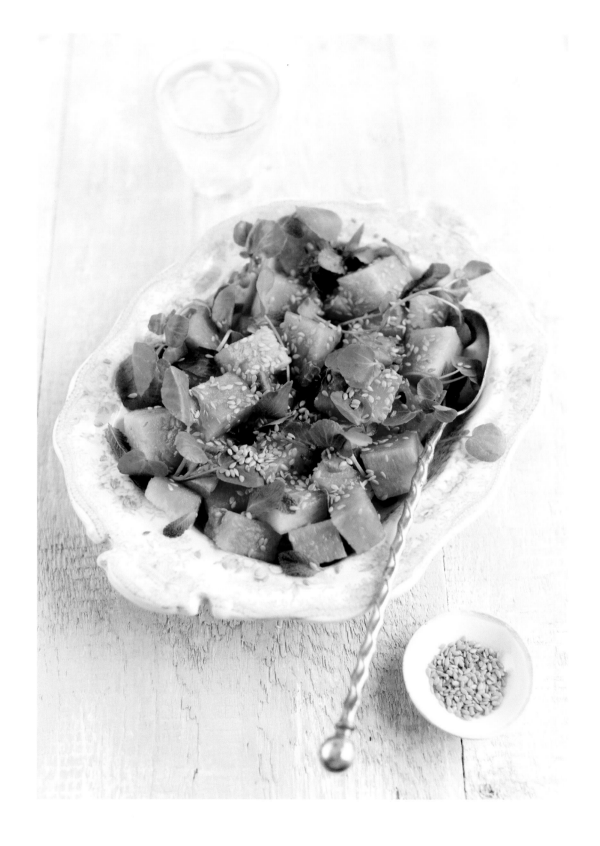

Fresh mint
petits pois

SERVES 2
AS A SIDE DISH

———

112 CALORIES
PER SERVING

———

FOR THE MINT SAUCE
- Handful of fresh mint, finely chopped
- 1 tbsp apple cider vinegar

- 1 tsp raw coconut oil
- 1 shallot, finely chopped
- 1 garlic clove, finely chopped
- 1 cup fresh or frozen petits pois or garden peas

If you haven't gathered already, I'm a big fan of mint – I find it complements all sorts of dishes, sweet or savory. This is my take on the classic side dish of minted peas – themselves a good source of vitamin C, which is essential for the production of collagen to support the structure of the skin. Peas are a summer crop, of course, so use fresh ones if you can.

1. Make the mint sauce by mixing together the fresh mint and apple cider vinegar in a bowl. Set aside.
2. Melt the oil in a large pan, then add the shallot and garlic and cook over medium heat for 3 minutes or until softened.
3. Meanwhile, steam or boil the peas in a medium saucepan of water for 2 minutes, then drain.
4. Add the mint sauce to the first pan, then mix in the peas and serve.

MINT APPETIZER
Eating mint before, rather than after, a meal activates the salivary glands, releasing digestive enzymes that help break down food.

Fennel and celery soup

SERVES 2

————

85 CALORIES
PER SERVING

————

- 1 tsp coconut oil
- 2 large garlic cloves, finely chopped
- 2 shallots, finely chopped
- 1 large fennel bulb, chopped, reserving the fronds to garnish
- 6 celery stalks, chopped
- Leaves from 2 sprigs of thyme
- ¾ cup chicken stock (to make your own, see p. 228)
- Juice of 1 lemon
- Sea salt and black pepper
- Flaxseed oil, to serve

I like having this when I've overindulged and am feeling bloated and uncomfortable. I make a big batch and freeze it. It's surprisingly filling and it works quickly to help soothe an upset tummy, reduce the appetite and aid detoxification, plus it tastes creamy and delicious. It's the ultimate weight-loss soup – you will wake up feeling skinny for sure!

1. Heat the coconut oil in a large saucepan over medium heat. Add the garlic, shallots, fennel, celery and thyme and cook for about 5 minutes or until the vegetables are soft and translucent. Season with a pinch of salt and pepper and continue to cook for a further minute.
2. Pour in the chicken stock and bring to a boil, then reduce the heat and simmer for 25 minutes.
3. Transfer the soup to a food processor and blend until smooth. Alternatively, use an immersion blender to whizz the mixture in the pan. Add the lemon juice.
4. Serve the soup garnished with the reserved fennel fronds and with a little flaxseed oil drizzled over.

FENNEL SEED TEA
Simply add 1 tablespoon of fennel seeds to a mug and fill with hot water.

Fig salad

———

230 CALORIES
PER SERVING

———

- 3½ oz burrata or buffalo mozzarella
- 2 fresh figs, quartered
- 2 large handfuls of arugula
- 1 tbsp extra-virgin olive oil
- 1 tbsp balsamic vinegar
- Fresh basil, to serve

Good for detoxifying the system, figs add a touch of natural sweetness, providing a healthier alternative to processed sugars, which can be detrimental to your skin.

1. Break the burrata or mozzarella into bite-sized pieces and place in a bowl with the figs. Add the arugula and mix well to make sure everything is evenly distributed.
2. Dress at the last minute, drizzling over the olive oil and balsamic vinegar in a zigzag motion, and scatter over basil leaves to serve.

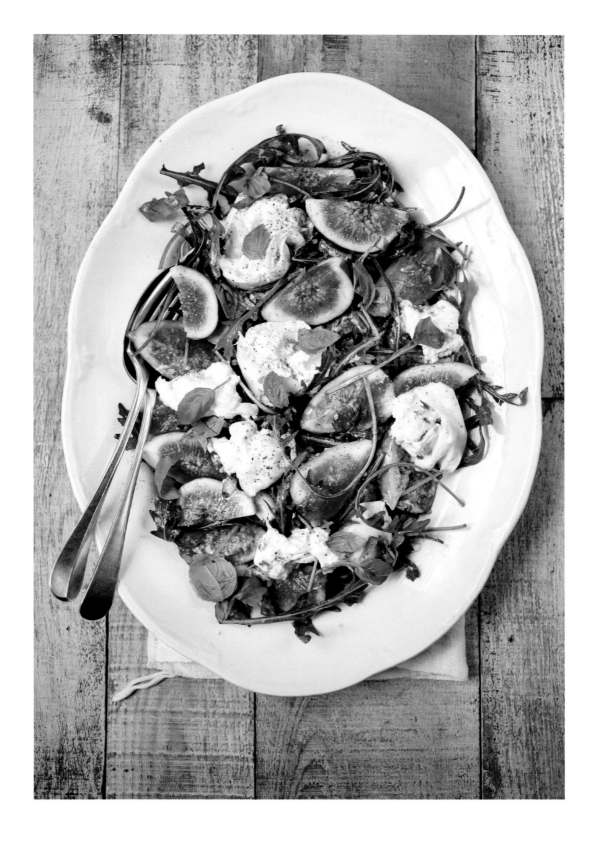

Alfalfa chicken pita

SERVES 2

———

444 CALORIES
PER SERVING

———

FOR THE MARINADE
- 2 tbsp ground cumin
- 1 tsp paprika
- 1 tsp ground cilantro
- 1 shallot, finely chopped
- 1 garlic clove,
  finely chopped
- Pinch of curry powder
- Juice of 1 lime
- 1 tbsp olive oil

- 2 large skinless and
  boneless chicken thighs
  or breasts
- 1 tbsp raw coconut oil

TO SERVE
- 1–2 slices of halloumi
- 1 gluten-free brown
  pita bread
- Handful of fresh
  cilantro, chopped
- Handful of alfalfa sprouts

Try alfalfa in this healthy but delicious lunch: alfalfa sprouts, with all their powerful nutrients, mixed with tasty cooked chicken (another food that's good for the skin – see p. 141) and grilled halloumi. Even the spices used for the marinade can benefit the skin: the antioxidant curcuminoids in turmeric (a component of curry powder), which give it the bright yellow color, may help inflammatory skin conditions such as psoriasis.

1. Mix all the marinade ingredients together in a bowl, then add the chicken thighs and leave to marinate in the fridge for 2 hours or overnight (or see tip).
2. Melt the coconut oil in a large skillet over high heat. When the pan is hot, add the marinated chicken thighs and cook on one side to brown the meat and seal in the spices before turning over to brown the other side. Fry for about 15 minutes in total or until the chicken is cooked through.
3. Shortly before the chicken has finished cooking, place the halloumi in the pan and cook for a couple of minutes on each side. Transfer the chicken and halloumi to a plate and cut the meat into smaller pieces.
4. To assemble, slice open the pita bread and fill it with the halloumi, chicken, cilantro and alfalfa sprouts. Cut the filled pita in half and serve with some tzatziki (see p. 162) on the side.

TIPS
- If you don't have time to leave the chicken to marinate, simply pop it into a resealable freezer bag with the marinade ingredients and squeeze everything together so that the chicken is well coated. You can then cook the chicken straight away.
- The chicken also tastes delicious served on its own with the Pomegranate Spring Salad on p. 74.

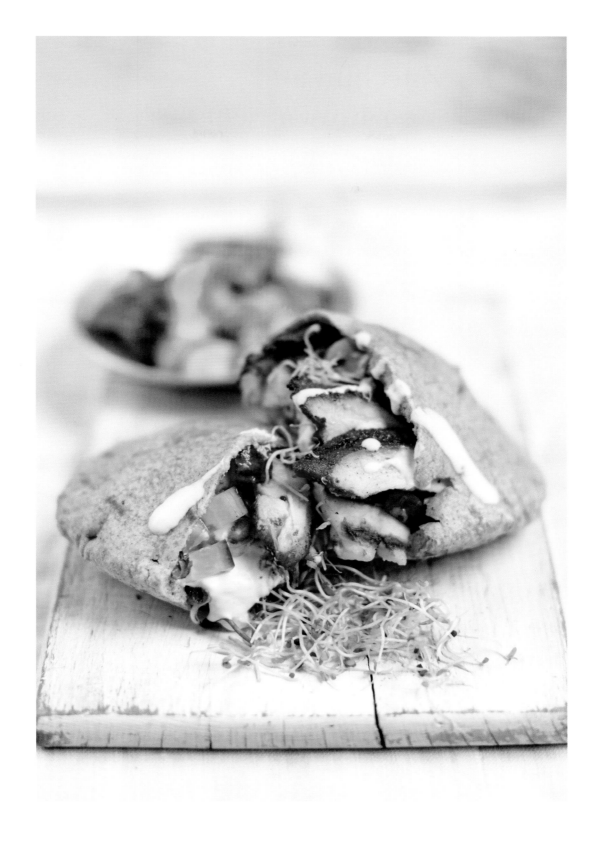

Zucchini and brown rice spaghetti

SERVES 2

———

469 CALORIES
PER SERVING

———

- 3 tbsp olive oil
- 3 oz dried brown rice spaghetti
- 2 shallots, finely chopped
- 3 garlic cloves, finely chopped
- 1 large zucchini, spiralized
- Handful of fresh flat-leaf parsley, finely chopped
- Finely grated zest of 1 lemon
- 1–2 fresh red chile, seeded and finely chopped
- Sea salt and black pepper
- 1 oz Parmesan cheese, grated, to serve

Zucchinis are tailor-made for using with a spiralizer to create zucchini noodles, or "zoodles." Unlike standard wheat pasta, you won't be left feeling bloated and overly full, so you can indulge to your heart's content! I first learned about zoodles from famous people that I've worked with who were trying to get in shape. I've actually added in a little cooked spaghetti to bulk out the dish, using brown rice spaghetti, which has the advantage of being gluten-free as well as a fantastic source of skin-boosting B vitamins. If you want to get skinny, simply omit the spaghetti; if you're hungry, keep it in. You do need a spiralizer for this recipe. If you don't have one, however, you can cut the zucchini into strips with a vegetable peeler or mandolin.

1. Add 1 tablespoon of olive oil and the brown rice spaghetti to a large pan of boiling water and cook according to the package instructions (about 12 minutes) or until tender. Drain the spaghetti in a colander and leave to sit for 1–2 minutes.
2. Meanwhile, heat 2 tablespoons of the olive oil in a large, deep-sided skillet or wok and add the shallots and garlic. Cook over medium heat for about 2 minutes or until soft.
3. Add the zucchini noodles and season with a little salt and pepper, then cover the pan with a lid and steam for 5 minutes.
4. Add the parsley, lemon zest and chile and remove from the heat.
5. Add the drained spaghetti to the saucepan and combine with the zucchini sauce.
6. Divide between plates and serve sprinkled with grated Parmesan.

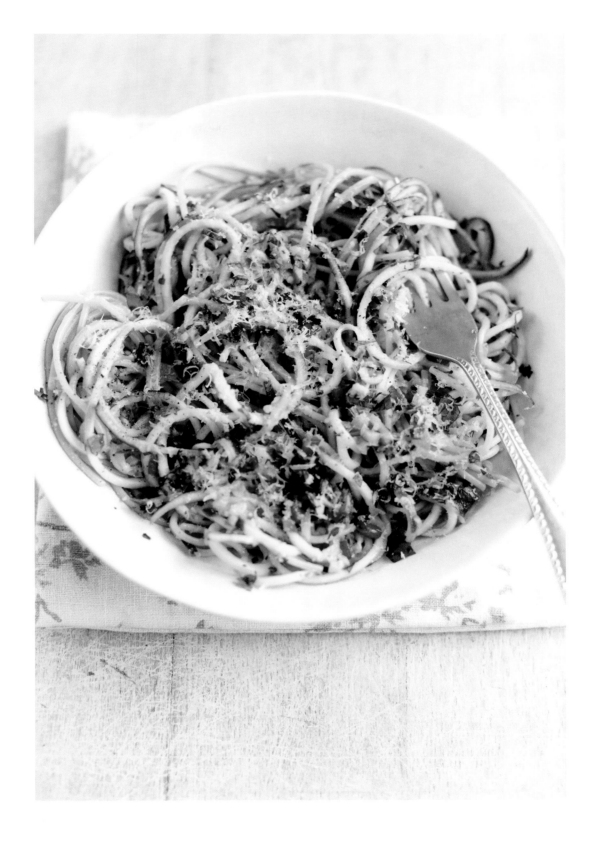

White fish with parsley butter

SERVES 2

———

350 CALORIES
PER SERVING

———

- 4 new potatoes, peeled (optional) and halved
- 4 Jerusalem artichokes, peeled and quartered
- 2 cod fillets
- 1 tbsp olive oil, plus extra for drizzling
- 1 cup rainbow chard
- 2 tsp butter
- ¾ oz flat-leaf parsley, finely chopped
- Sea salt and black pepper
- ½ lemon, cut in half, to serve

For me, parsley is a sentimental ingredient as it reminds me of my mum's cooking – it was something she loved to grow in the garden; I naturally associate it with home-cooked dishes as a result. This recipe must be my favorite from my mum's repertoire – flaky white fish (also good for the skin – see p. 207) and a buttery parsley sauce, which she would serve with new potatoes and peas. I've tried to update the sauce to make it healthier and less time consuming by cutting out the flour and cream from the original. I use tons of parsley now that I know it is a wonder herb: I put it in salads and soups and stir it into mash.

1. Preheat the oven to 350°F.
2. Fill a large pan with water, add the potatoes and artichokes and boil for 15 minutes or until tender.
3. Meanwhile, place the cod in the middle of a sheet of foil, brush with oil and season with salt and pepper.
4. Fold over the edges of the foil to wrap up the fish, scrunching up the open ends to form a boat-shaped parcel, and transfer to a baking sheet. Place in the oven to bake for about 12 minutes or until tender. (Leave wrapped in foil until ready to serve.)
5. Drain the potatoes and Jerusalem artichokes in a colander and then place back in the saucepan, drizzle with olive oil and season with salt and pepper. Put a lid on the pan and shake vigorously. Remove the lid and then use a potato masher or fork to flatten slightly or roughly mash. Set aside in the pan to keep warm.
6. Place the chard in a colander and pour over boiling water to soften.
7. Melt the butter in a small saucepan and add the parsley, then remove from the heat and stir together.
8. Divide the blanched chard and mash between plates and add a fillet of cod to each. Spoon a little of the fish cooking juices over the cod and serve with the parsley butter and a wedge of lemon.

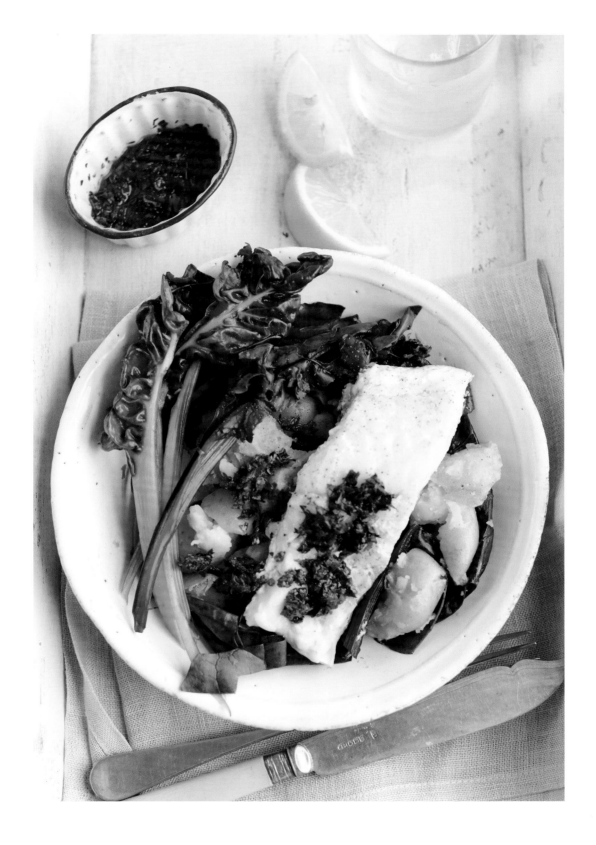

Brown stew chicken with black-eyed pea rice

SERVES 2

————

700 CALORIES
PER SERVING

————

FOR THE CHICKEN STEW
- 4 skinless and boneless chicken thighs
- Juice of 1 lemon
- 2 tsp curry powder
- 1 tsp ground allspice
- Pinch of crushed dried chiles
- 1 tbsp raw coconut oil
- 1 vegetable stock cube
- 1½ cups boiling water
- 1 onion, chopped
- 2 garlic cloves, crushed
- 2 fresh tomatoes, roughly chopped, or a 14½-oz can of organic chopped tomatoes
- Sprig of thyme
- 1 fresh Scotch bonnet chile pepper
- Sea salt and black pepper

FOR THE RICE
- ¾ cup brown rice, well rinsed
- 1 onion, chopped
- 2 garlic cloves, crushed
- 15-oz can of black-eyed peas, drained and rinsed
- 1 tsp butter
- Sprig of thyme

I love cooking Jamaican food and to get this recipe I had to beg because my friend Earl – an excellent cook, if better known as a hairstylist to the stars – doesn't give up his culinary secrets easily. Whenever I have a dinner party and want to cook Caribbean food, I get Earl to come over earlier to help me. This stew needs time and TLC, but it's well worth it. Keep the Scotch bonnet chile whole and remove before serving – this will just add flavor, not heat or spice.

1. Preheat the oven to 400°F.
2. Place the chicken in a bowl, pour in the lemon juice and 1 cup of cold water and leave in the fridge to marinate for 20 minutes.
3. Remove the chicken from the fridge and drain off the marinating water. Rinse the chicken in fresh water and add to the empty bowl with the curry powder, allspice and crushed chiles, seasoning with salt and pepper. Massage into the meat.
4. Add the coconut oil to a deep roasting pan or heatproof casserole dish and place in the oven for 5 minutes to heat up. Remove the pan from the oven (the oil should be really hot) and carefully add the spice-coated chicken before placing the pan back in the oven.
5. Cook the chicken for about 30 minutes, turning occasionally during the first 5 minutes to seal each side and brown. When cooked, the chicken should be a rich dark brown in color.
6. Meanwhile, place the stock cube in a jar, pour in the boiling water and stir to dissolve.
7. Remove the chicken from the oven and transfer to a medium saucepan if you used a roasting pan. Set on the burner over high heat and add the onion, garlic, tomatoes and stock. Bring to a boil, then reduce the heat to a low simmer. Add the thyme and Scotch bonnet, place a lid on the pan and leave to cook for about 50 minutes over very low heat, topping up with a splash of water as needed.
8. After the chicken has been cooking for about 30 minutes, tip the rice into another medium saucepan; add the onion and garlic and enough water to cover by about ½ inch.

    BLACK-EYED PEA (P. 87)

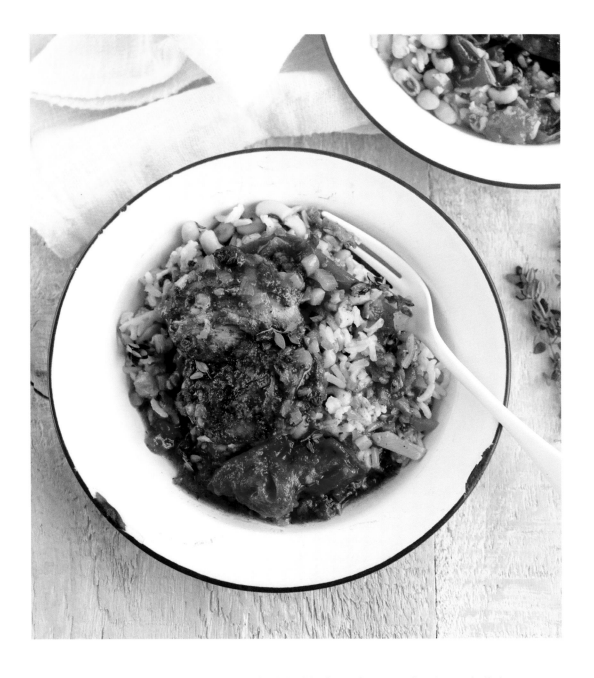

9. Add the black-eyed peas to the rice and stir to combine, then add the butter and sprig of thyme. Bring the rice mixture to the boil, then turn down the heat to a gentle simmer and place a lid on the pan. Cook for 20 minutes or until the rice is tender and has absorbed all the liquid. Check for seasoning.
10. Discard the thyme and Scotch bonnet from the stew. Serve the stew with the black-eyed pea rice.

Spicy fish
with limes

SERVES 2

————

265 CALORIES
PER SERVING

————

- 1 whole fish (such as
  red snapper or sea bass),
  gutted and cleaned
  (see tip below)
- 1 fresh red chile,
  seeded and finely chopped
- 1 tbsp honey
- 1 garlic clove, finely
  chopped
- Handful of fresh cilantro,
  finely chopped
- 1 shallot, finely chopped
- Juice of 1 lime
- Sea salt

FOR THE SALAD
- Handful of arugula
- 1 small cucumber, chopped
- Juice of 1 lemon

I was inspired to make this recipe after many trips to
Thailand – a place I love to visit. It's such an easy dish,
and so light, fresh and clean-tasting, with added benefits
to the skin from the fish, cilantro and cucumber. Squeeze
a generous amount of lime juice on to the fish, safe in the
knowledge that your skin will be reaping all the rewards.

1. Preheat the oven to 350°F.
2. Score the skin of the fish diagonally a few times with
    a sharp knife and rub sea salt into the skin.
3. Combine the chile, honey, garlic, shallot, cilantro and
    lime juice in a small bowl and rub this mixture over the
    fish, inside and out.
4. Place the fish in the middle of a large piece of
    parchment paper or foil. Fold the paper or foil over
    the fish as though wrapping a present, scrunching up
    the open edges at either end to create a boat-shaped
    parcel.
5. Place the wrapped fish on a baking sheet and cook in
    the oven for 20 minutes or until tender.
6. Meanwhile, combine the arugula, cucumber and
    lemon juice in a bowl.
7. To serve, fillet the top layer of cooked fish and transfer
    to a plate, then carefully pull away the fish bone and
    head before transferring the rest of the filleted fish to
    the second plate. Serve with the salad.

TIPS
- Ask your fishmonger to gut and clean the fish for you,
  or, if you prefer, simply substitute with four fillets.
- This can also be cooked in foil on a barbecue.

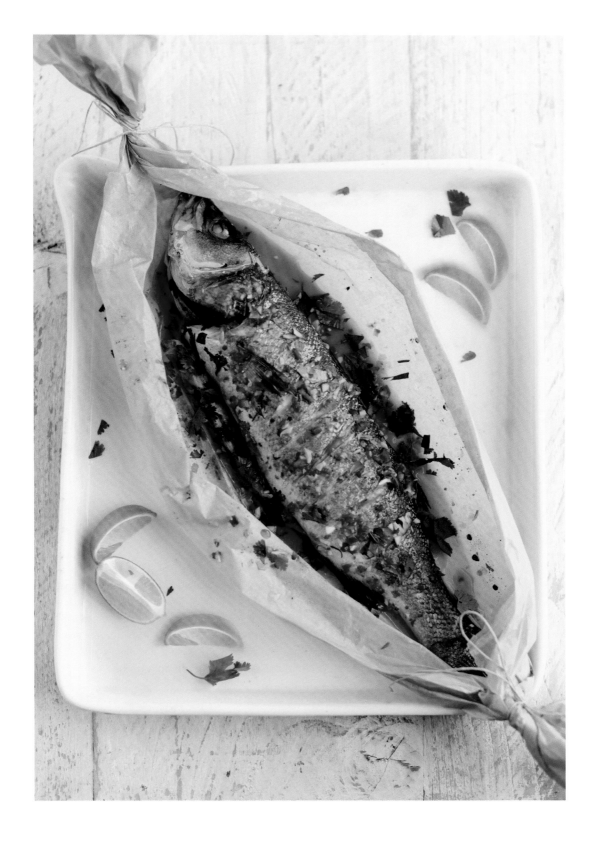

Cucumber and mango salsa

SERVES 2

————

102 CALORIES
PER SERVING

————

- Flesh of 1 mango, finely diced
- ½ cucumber, finely diced
- 4 scallions, finely chopped
- Small bunch of fresh mint, finely chopped
- Small bunch of fresh cilantro, finely chopped
- Juice of ½ lime
- 1 tbsp sunflower seeds, to serve

I like anything with cucumber in it, from juices, salads and crudités to an ice-cold glass of Pimm's. Being a Brit, I naturally fancy a cucumber sandwich from time to time, too. This recipe makes such a refreshing accompaniment to a main dish on a summer day – it goes with just about any meal you can think of. Light and fresh, it's perfect with wild rice salads (see p. 106) or curries, for instance; the sweetness of the mango and juicy crunch of the cucumber complementing any spiciness. The mint, cilantro and lime in this dish have skin-benefiting qualities, too.

1. Add the mango and cucumber to a bowl with the scallions, herbs and lime juice and toss together.
2. Divide between plates and sprinkle with the sunflower seeds to serve.

Iced white tea

SERVES 4

————

0 CALORIES
PER SERVING

————

- 4 white tea bags
- 1 lime, chopped
- Handful of fresh mint, chopped, plus fresh sprigs to serve
- Ice cubes

I love to make up a pitcher of white tea with ice cubes and some tangy limes and mint – both skin-benefiting ingredients (see pp. 93 and 94) – as a refreshing summer alternative to aging sugar-laden concoctions. It's a great choice, too, if you're not drinking alcohol but others around you are. Fill a glass with this delicious iced tea and you won't feel at all that you're missing out on the festivities.

1. Place the tea bags in a teapot and pour over a kettle of freshly boiled water. Allow it to brew for a few minutes before pouring into a pitcher and allowing to cool.
2. Add the lime, mint and a handful of ice cubes and chill in the fridge.
3. To serve, pour into glasses and serve with extra ice cubes and a sprig of mint added to each glass.

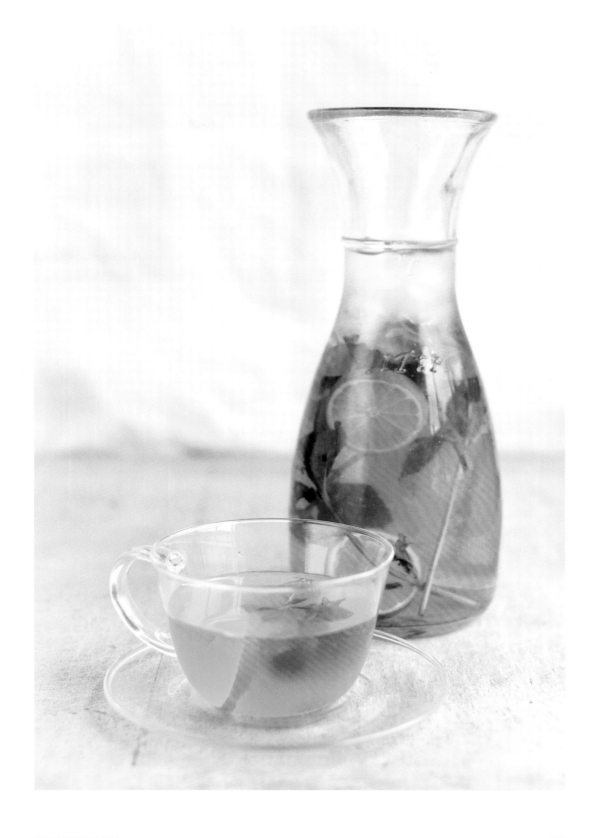

Strawberry salad with balsamic vinegar and fresh mint

SERVES 4

———

27 CALORIES
PER SERVING

———

- 14 oz ripe strawberries, hulled and sliced
- Squeeze of lemon juice
- Handful of mint, finely chopped
- 1 tsp aged balsamic vinegar
- 1 tsp Stevia (optional)

TO SERVE (OPTIONAL)
- Cream or ice cream
- Balsamic vinegar

Of course, no one really needs any encouragement to eat strawberries because they're so tasty just as they are, but their natural sweetness makes them perfect for desserts, as you don't have to add extra sugar—ideal for when you're trying to quit or phase out refined sugars but still have a craving. A single serving of this healthy dessert provides an entire day's worth of vitamin C!

1. Place all the ingredients in a bowl and toss together until the strawberries are coated with the lemon juice and mint.
2. Serve immediately with fresh cream or ice cream and a drizzle of balsamic vinegar, if desired.

MIXED BERRIES
All berries – raspberries, blueberries, blackberries and blackcurrants, as well as strawberries – are brilliant for feeding the skin, and it's good to have a mixture as the different colors each denote a different type of antioxidant.

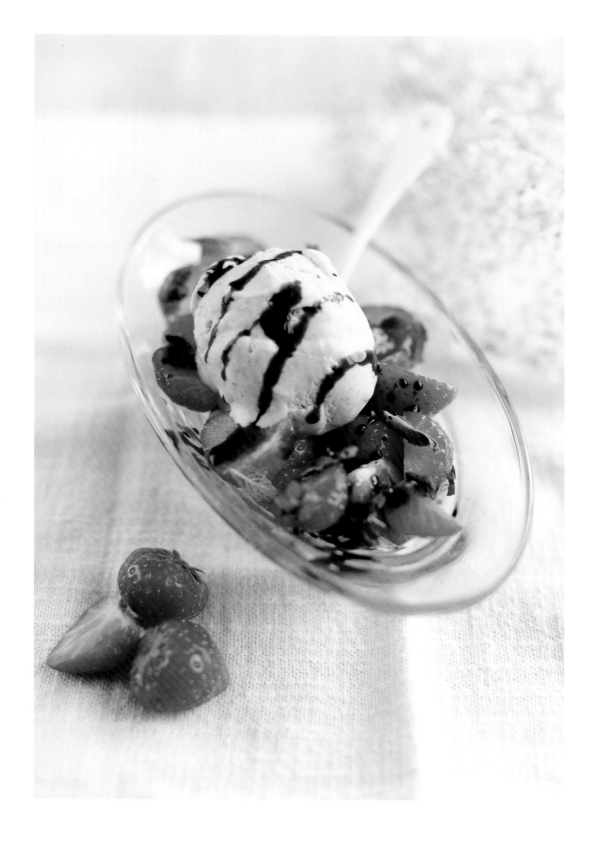

Frozen banana ice pops

MAKES 6 ICE POPS

————

102 CALORIES
PER SERVING

————

- 1¾ cups coconut or unsweetened almond milk
- 2 large bananas, peeled
- 2 tbsp runny honey
- 1 tsp vanilla extract
- 1 tbsp shredded coconut
- Handful of ground hazelnuts (or extra shredded coconut), for dipping

If I'm in a rush in the morning and need something a little more substantial, I always reach for a banana – they're great for kick-starting the system. I don't eat them much otherwise, but if I'm starving and can't be bothered cooking, a banana really does the trick. This frozen mixture of mashed-up banana, coconut cream and honey makes a gorgeously creamy treat during the summer months. It's just as sweet as a commercial ice pop but with a natural and interesting flavor with a host of skin-feeding actives as well. The vanilla extract and coconut add sweetness, making a good alternative to sugar, which can affect the health of your skin if you consume too much (see p. 16). These are great for when you want to show off for your guests!

1. Pour half of the milk into a food processor and add the bananas, honey and ½ teaspoon of vanilla extract, then process until smooth.
2. In a bowl, whisk together the remaining coconut milk and vanilla extract.
3. Divide the banana mixture between six ice pop molds.
4. Layer the coconut mixture on top of the banana mixture, then leave in the freezer for at least 6 hours or until completely frozen.
5. Remove the ice pops from their molds by dipping them in warm water for 10 seconds. Tip the ground hazelnuts (or shredded coconut) into a deep bowl, then dip the top 2–3 inches of each ice pop into the nuts to coat.
6. Place the ice pops back in the freezer to set. They will be ready after 5 minutes or whenever you fancy one.

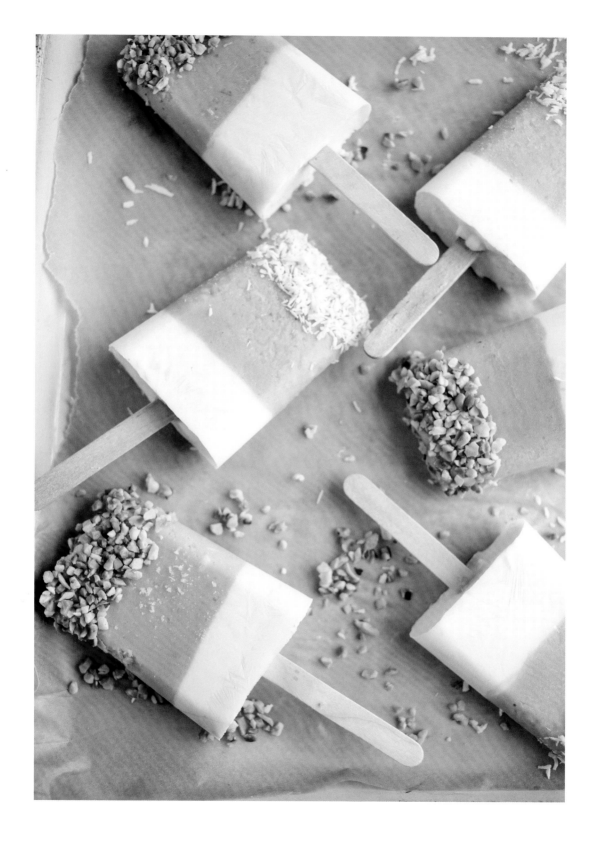

Perfumed chocolates

MAKES
20—24 CHOCOLATES

————

180 CALORIES
PER CHOCOLATE

————

FOR THE ALMOND PASTE
- ½ cup blanched almonds
- 3 tbsp unsweetened desiccated coconut
- 1 tbsp coconut oil
- 2 tbsp Xylitol

- 8 oz raw cocoa butter
- 12 tbsp raw cacao (or cocoa) powder
- 3 tbsp maple syrup
- 1½ tsp lavender or rose essence

TO DECORATE (OPTIONAL)
- Edible flowers
- Fresh mint leaves

It may seem a little bit "old lady" to make perfumed sweets, but these are a show-stopper. They are time-consuming, but well worth all the effort as your friends will be impressed. They quite rich, too, so good for sharing. I like to decorate them with fresh flowers from the garden as a finishing touch. These are a good example of how a treat can be healthy for you too. Surprisingly, each chocolate provides 10% of your recommended daily allowance of iron and 20% of your magnesium, and mood- and skin-enhancing properties!

1. First make the almond paste. Place the nuts in a bowl, cover with water and leave to soak for 1 hour. Drain and then add to a food processor with the desiccated coconut, coconut oil and Xylitol. Blend to a paste.
2. Use the paste to fill 20–24 holes of a silicone ice-cube tray, then place in the freezer to set for 1 hour.
3. Place the cocoa butter in a medium heatproof bowl and set over a medium saucepan of gently simmering water. (The base of the bowl shouldn't touch the water in the pan.) When the cocoa butter has melted, remove from the heat and leave to cool for 10 minutes (still in the bowl over the pan), then mix in the cacao/cocoa powder, maple syrup and lavender or rose essence.
4. Leave the mixture to cool down further until thick enough to coat the back of a spoon.
5. Remove the lumps of paste from the ice-cube tray and, using a spoon and fork, dip each into the perfumed chocolate, then carefully lift out and place on a sheet lined with parchment paper. When all the fillings have been coated, place in the freezer to set for 15 minutes.
6. Repeat this process twice more, so that each filling is covered in three layers of chocolate (see tip below). Store in the freezer.
7. Serve, decorated with flowers or mint, if you like.

TIP
- Kept in the bowl over the saucepan, the chocolate should remain runny. If it does set, however, simply place back over the heat.
- Any leftover chocolate is divine drizzled over berries and ice cream and served with a sprig of fresh mint.

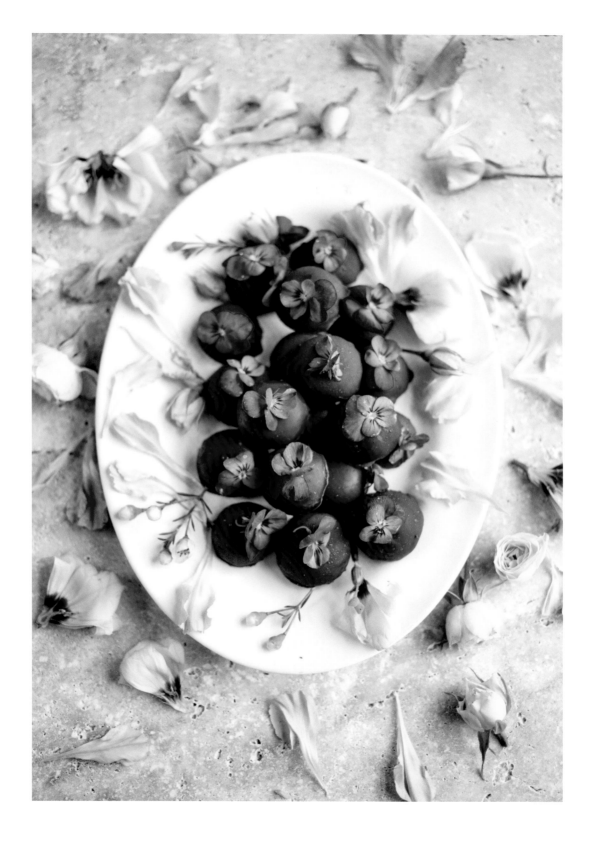

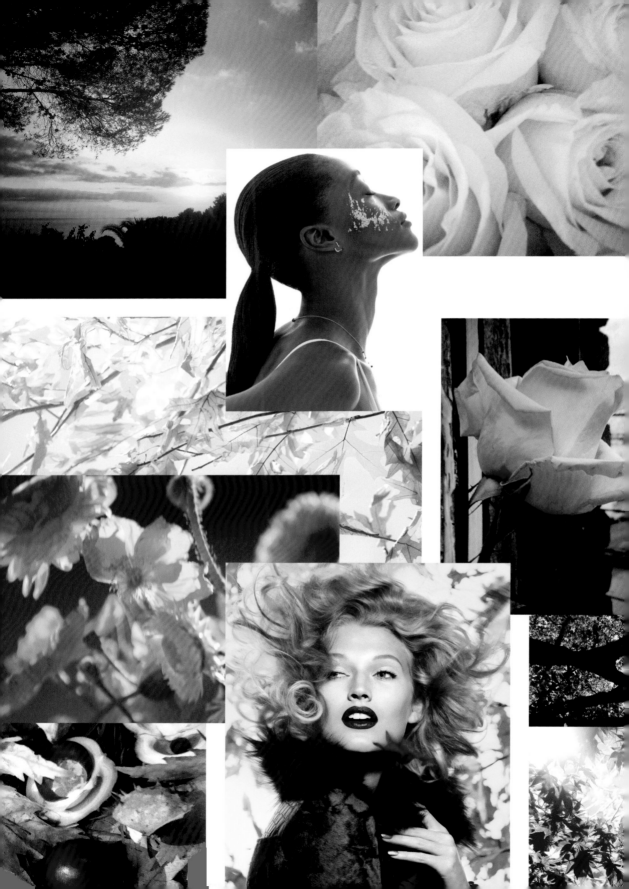

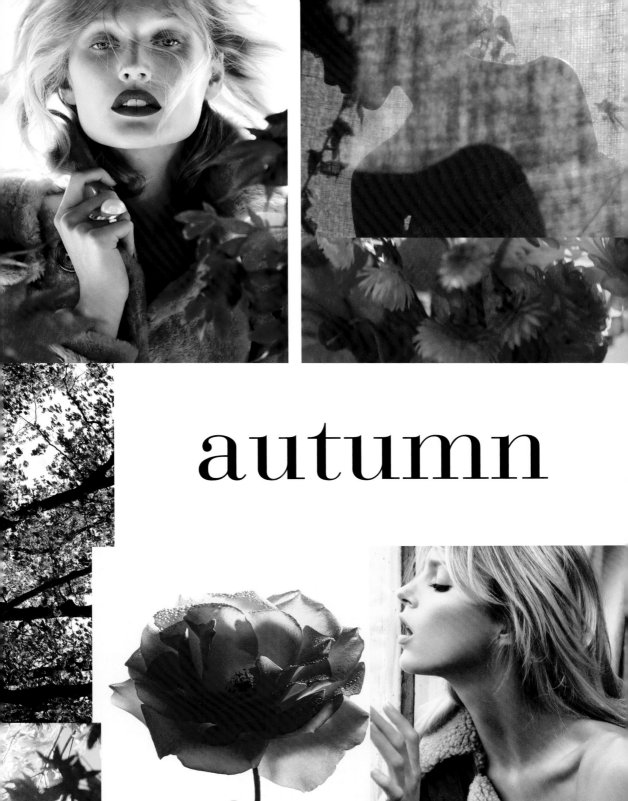

autumn

A time to prepare

I tend to equate autumn with the new fashion season – for spring and summer the following year! That's because the fashion industry works six months in advance, shooting in the autumn for collections to be advertized in the New Year. A period of transition, it is the perfect time to prepare for the colder months. Post-summer, the skin needs some TLC – especially purifying and replenishing treatments. It can feel dull and dehydrated and in need of a good dose of moisture in preparation for winter's environmental aggressors – cold weather and central heating being the chief culprits.

As it turns colder, I look to slightly richer skincare formulas – creamier cleansers and more intensive moisturizers and other treatments.

Try to consume a range of good oils to provide hydration from within – think coconut oil and foods with omega-3 essential fatty acids. Foods rich in selenium will help address any damage from too much summer sun, as will foods containing vitamins A, C and E. Autumn is also a time to ensure your immune system is in good working order. Stock up on foods that help keep colds and flu at bay, such as garlic and ginger, and dose up on echinacea and lots of water.

Don't forget to exercise now it's becoming colder; getting in at least one 20-minute walk a day will help you attain a good night's sleep. Often it's not just about going to bed early; it's about ensuring you get a good night's sleep by exercising, meditating and eating well (and not too late).

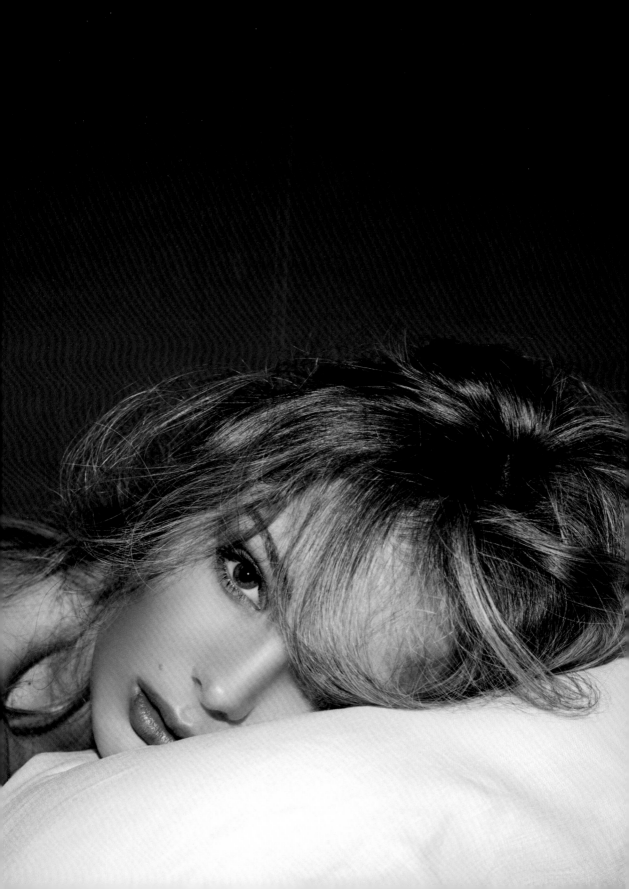

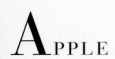APPLE

An apple a day keeps the doctor away, or so they say. But is it just an old wives' tale? Apparently not! Known in Ayurvedic terms for their ability to cool the body after the summer, thanks to their anti-inflammatory qualities, apples are a bit of an unsung hero when it comes to health and beauty. They're full of fiber, which of course helps keep things moving in the digestive system, keeping the colon clear and the skin glowing with good health while also helping you to feel fuller for longer. Don't be fooled into drinking apple juice: with no roughage to slow down the impact of all the sugar it contains, it won't have the same effect at all. The skin of apples contains the pigment quercetin, which acts as a powerful anti-aging compound, helping to offset the damage caused by UV radiation, so it's important to always eat the apple skin to ensure you're getting the full complement of skin-benefiting nutrients. In addition, the copper in apples helps in the production of melanin in the body – the pigment that colors your skin and protects from the sun. Containing vitamin C, apples help both to boost the immune system – a great thing for autumn, when the flu season first appears – and brighten the complexion by helping to synthesize collagen for a more youthful complexion.

SKIN-FEEDING NUTRIENTS

- Dietary fiber:
  pectin
- Minerals:
  copper
- Phytochemicals:
  flavonoids
    (ellagic acid,
    quercetin)

- Vitamins:
  A
  B5 (pantothenic acid)
  B9 (folate)
  C

STEWED APPLES WITH CINNAMON (P. 180)

BEEF

THE IRON BOOSTER

I don't eat a lot of meat as a rule, and when I do, I tend to go for chicken or fish; red meat is not usually my thing. That said, I recognize when my body feels like it's running on empty, and often it's a lack of iron that's at the root of it. As women, we're prone to iron deficiency due to our monthly cycle – the blood loss can make us feel run down and lethargic with a pale, lifeless complexion. I'm not rigid in my approach to food, but I try to listen to my body and eat according to the season whenever I can, and a bit of red meat is sometimes the very thing I need. I try to eat organic, grass-fed beef because it's hormone- and antibiotic-free – plus the animal will have had a better quality of life – and I know the meat will be both tasty and loaded with nutrients. Packed with iron and protein, which both boost energy and promote general well-being, beef also helps to keep the skin looking lustrous and your hair thick and glossy. Brimming with a range of B vitamins, beef also helps improve mood, maintains good circulation and supports the skin, aiding cell regeneration. So if, like me, you choose to eat red meat on occasion, it's good to opt for an ethically reared, premium-quality piece of beef that you can be sure will contain a fine array of nutrients to help build you up for the colder months ahead.

SKIN-FEEDING NUTRIENTS

- Minerals:
  copper
  magnesium
  manganese
  phosphorus
  potassium
  selenium
  zinc
- Protein:
  all nine essential
    amino acids

- Vitamins:
  B1 (thiamine)
  B2 (riboflavin)
  B3 (niacin)
  B5 (pantothenic acid)
  B6 (pyroxidine)
  B9 (folate)
  B12 (cobalamin)
  D
  E

MEATBALLS ARRABBIATA (P. 174)

BROWN RICE

THE LOW-GI WHOLE FOOD

Did you know that brown rice is the same grain as white rice, just less processed? Only the outermost layer – the hull – is removed in the production of brown rice, leaving the nutrient-rich outer layers, which is why brown rice is darker and tougher than its white counterpart. I love cooking with it, not just because it's superior nutritionally to white rice, but because I prefer the nutty flavor and the fact that you need to eat less of it in order to feel full. Known as a low-glycemic superfood, brown rice releases its energy slowly, meaning the body is not knocked around by the blood-sugar highs and lows that you get from consuming the simpler carbohydrates in more refined foodstuffs (such as white rice, bread and other baked goods). This slow-burning, low-GI approach to eating is not only good for the skin – blood-sugar spikes having an aging effect, by contrast – but it's also excellent for the metabolism, promoting weight loss and bowel regularity, which make it the perfect all-arounder. Brown rice is also high in fiber, so it tends to pull everything with it through the digestive tract, keeping the intestines clear and allowing other nutrients to be absorbed more easily – including all the wonderful skin-benefiting vitamins and minerals listed below.

SKIN-FEEDING NUTRIENTS

- Dietary fiber
- Minerals:
  calcium
  iron
  magnesium
  manganese
  phosphorus
  potassium
  selenium
- Protein
- Vitamins:
  B1 (thiamine)
  B3 (niacin)
  B9 (folate)
  E

BROWN RICE AND VEGETABLE PILAF (P. 172)

THE LEAN PROTEIN

CHICKEN

Apart from its great flavor and versatility, I find chicken the easiest meat to digest and the best for keeping me feeling fuller for longer. Unlike some other meats, chicken doesn't cause inflammation in the body when you digest it, so it's a great source of lean, low-fat protein – plus it contains a host of nutrients that feed the skin. It's really important to choose organic, free-range chicken. Intensively farmed poultry is hugely toxic to the body and skin due to the chemical additives in the chicken feed; buying organic chicken is a better ethical choice, too. Chicken has high levels of selenium, which helps repair sun damage to the skin, including unwanted pigmentation. Helping to promote muscle growth and development due to its high protein content, as well as being so lean, chicken is a great option for those watching their weight. High in an essential amino acid called tryptophan – which can't be produced by the body and so must be obtained through the diet – chicken is perfect for when you're feeling a bit low. This is because tryptophan is needed to produce serotonin in the brain, the "feel-good" hormone that helps you contend with stress – always bad news for the skin – enhancing overall feelings of well-being and helping you to sleep. That's why they give you chicken soup when you're ill (see my Hearty Chicken Soup on p. 218). The benefits of chicken don't end there: it's also a rich source of phosphorus, promoting strong bones and teeth, and potassium, a mineral that helps with fluid retention and blood pressure – another stress-busting nutrient and hence great for the skin.

SKIN-FEEDING NUTRIENTS

- Minerals:
  copper
  iron
  magnesium
  phosphorus
  potassium
  selenium
  zinc
- Protein:
  all nine essential
    amino acids

- Vitamins:
  B3 (niacin)
  B5 (pantothenic
  acid)
  B9 (folate)
  choline

CHICKPEA

Chickpeas weren't a food I grew up with; I was introduced to them when spending time in North Africa in my early twenties. I enjoyed the nutty taste and how they filled me up but without costing much – perfect for anyone on a budget. I also loved the way the chickpeas took on the flavor of the dish – so spicy and full of Eastern promise. If you're trying to stay away from refined sugars, chickpeas make a good alternative to carbs like pasta because of their low-glycemic profile. What this means in real terms is that they're so rich in protein and fiber that the energy released is slow-burning, so you will feel fuller for longer and will suffer fewer peaks and troughs in energy levels. For skin, it's hugely important to keep your blood sugar on an even keel. When you eat simple carbohydrates and refined sugars, your blood sugar rapidly increases, causing the body to produce insulin spikes in response; this can lead to acne-causing hormonal changes and general inflammation. For anyone suffering from acne or "angry" skin conditions, it's a good idea to consider low-GI options like chickpeas for this reason.

SKIN-FEEDING NUTRIENTS

- Dietary fiber
- Fatty acids: omega-3
- Minerals: calcium iron manganese phosphorus
- Phytochemicals: saponins
- Protein: amino acids (tryptophan)
- Vitamins: B9 (folate)

CHICKPEA AND CHICKEN TAGINE (P. 162)

CHILE

THE CIRCULATION BOOSTER

Chiles have been used across cultures and throughout time, not just for their fiery flavor-enhancing properties, but for their medicinal effect on the body, too. Full of a powerful active called capsaicin – which is what gives chiles their spicy taste – they're known for their ability to reduce blood pressure and improve circulation by encouraging the blood vessels to relax and dilate. Although it's counter-intuitive given how fiery they are, chiles are actually anti-inflammatory, making them hugely helpful for treating conditions like psoriasis and arthritis (although those suffering from rosacea might want to tread with caution, as spicy foods are known to aggravate this condition). And even if you don't have a specific skin condition, chiles will help keep your complexion looking fresh and uncongested. Although there are no foods that can trigger weight loss or have a significant impact on their own, chiles may help boost the metabolism and circulation by activating receptors in the body which set off the process of energy burning, making them a great addition to any dish as part of a healthy weight-loss diet and exercise program. I don't need any encouragement to eat more chiles – I love spicy foods – so adding a bit to most savory dishes is a no-brainer for me.

SKIN-FEEDING NUTRIENTS

- Dietary fiber
- Minerals:
  copper
  iron
  magnesium
  manganese
  potassium
- Phytochemicals:
  capsaicin
  carotenoids
  (alpha- and
  beta-carotene,
  cryptoxanthin,
  lutein,
  zeaxanthin)
- Vitamins:
  A
  B1 (thiamine)
  B2 (riboflavin)
  B3 (niacin)
  B6 (pyridoxine)
  C

STICKY CHILE BEEF (P. 170)   143

COCONUT WATER

If you didn't know already, I'm a massive fan of raw coconut water. I can't emphasize enough just how potent it is as a beautifier for the skin – and hence an essential addition to any skin-boosting regimen. It's also the best post-workout drink there is: a good balance of electrolytes (including calcium, magnesium and potassium), it works to replace lost fluids and salts in minutes, much more effectively than any commercially produced drink. Coconut water can't be in a carton; it needs to be in a refrigerated bottle (like milk) and it needs to be organic. Its rich vitamin content (mostly B and C) works to create that expensive-looking glow we're all chasing, plus coconut water is known to be helpful in treating stress and depression, both of which can adversely affect the skin. It also works to boost your metabolism and reduce bloating – ideal for anyone on a fitness kick or who suffers from digestive problems like IBS. A diuretic, coconut water helps speed up the elimination of toxins, and it helps to regulate blood sugar, making it an excellent choice for diabetics or anyone with blood-sugar issues. I've said it countless times, but there is literally no way for skin to look radiant if it's dehydrated – coconut water helps to address this, rehydrating the body on every level and helping to keep the connective tissue, including collagen in the skin, hydrated and strong. Coconut water contains nutrients that work to support cell growth and turnover for a younger-looking complexion, while anti-inflammatory phytochemicals help to regulate the body's pH levels for a clearer, less breakout-prone skin.

SKIN-FEEDING NUTRIENTS

- Minerals:
  calcium
  chloride
  magnesium
  manganese
  potassium
  zinc
- Phytochemicals
- Probiotics
- Vitamins:
  B1 (thiamine)
  B2 (riboflavin)
  B6 (pyridoxine)
  B9 (folate)
  C

GREEN PROTEIN SMOOTHIE (P. 156)

THE HEALTHY SUGAR ALTERNATIVE

D ATE

I have to admit that I ignored dates for most of my life until I lived in New York and started working with loads of supermodels, who were forever making smoothies. They'd tell me their recipes and mention that they added one date to the mix. It was always just one date. So, in the interest of doing anything to look as svelte as they did, I gave it a go and, to my astonishment, I found it was actually really sweet. I tried putting dates into other recipes and found the same thing: one date made the whole recipe sweet! It's incredible that these dried fruits are packed with so much sweetness through natural sugars. For any ex-sugar addicts, like me, or anyone who's trying to phase out refined sugar, dates are a brilliant natural alternative, packed with flavor but with less of a blood-sugar impact and hence less damaging to the skin. It should be said that all naturally sweet foods affect blood-sugar levels, including otherwise healthy foods like dates, which consist of almost 70 percent sugar. They should always be eaten in moderation and as a treat. However, while refined sugars do nothing for us nutritionally and are "empty" calories, dates are packed with fiber and contain minerals and vitamins with antioxidative properties that benefit the body and the skin. Nutrients include vitamin C, considered the anti-aging darling of the vitamin world, helping to brighten and support the collagen production for younger, wrinkle-free skin. Dates are also a source of vitamin B, which is great for treating various skin disorders, helping to repair and strengthen skin cells.

SKIN-FEEDING NUTRIENTS

- Dietary fiber
- Minerals:
  calcium
  iron
  magnesium
  phosphorus
  potassium

- Vitamins:
  B1 (thiamine)
  B2 (riboflavin)
  B3 (niacin)
  B5 (pantothenic acid)
  C

G ARLIC

THE ALL-AROUNDER

What can't garlic do? To me, the word "garlic" is synonymous with flavor – it forms the basis of so many dishes from so many cultures, as well as being widely recognized for its healing powers. Garlic is full of a natural chemical called allicin, which reacts with the blood when ingested to kill off harmful bacteria and viruses in the body, including those that cause skin conditions and infections. It can also work to kill the overgrowth in the gut of a fungus known as Candida albicans, a common problem that can be caused by overuse of antibiotics, poor diet or stress, among other things, and which is believed by some to be responsible for a range of health problems, including acne and other skin conditions. Containing a potent combination of antioxidants, which are hugely beneficial to the skin, and coupled with its antibiotic, antifungal properties, garlic helps to purify the blood, strengthen the immune system and boost circulation. The high levels of vitamin C work to stimulate the immune system, too: adding garlic to lemon, ginger and hot water is great for a cold. Garlic is also a rich source of sulfur, which is essential for the structure of skin, working with collagen to provide support. I could go on for ages about my love for this wondrous bulb, so if you don't already include it in your everyday cooking, perhaps its skin-purifying properties might convince you to do so. I always choose organically grown garlic that has a pinkish tinge to it, because that's how the Italians identify the best bulbs, and they should know because they use garlic in just about everything!

SKIN-FEEDING NUTRIENTS

- Dietary fiber
- Minerals:
  calcium
  copper
  iron
  magnesium
  manganese
  phosphorus
  potassium
  selenium
  sulfur
  zinc
- Phytochemicals:
  allicin
- Vitamins:
  B1 (thiamine)
  B2 (riboflavin)
  B3 (niacin)
  B6 (pyridoxine)
  B9 (folate)
  choline
  C

ROASTED GARLIC SPREAD (P. 168)

GHEE

It seems most cultures have their beauty cure-all: in Greece it's olive oil, in the Middle East it's argan oil – and in India it's ghee. Ghee is butter that's been clarified – melted down and its milk solids and any impurities removed, leaving just the refined fat. It's been used for centuries in India in cooking, medicine and skincare. Easy to digest and great for cooking because of the stability of its chemical structure, even at a high temperature, ghee should be a staple in everyone's kitchen cupboard. (As long as it's kept in an airtight container, it doesn't even need to be refrigerated!) Clarifying butter removes the protein (casein) and sugar (lactose), making ghee a pure fat that's super easy to digest, even by those who are lactose-intolerant. Ghee is wonderful for the skin and general health, too. Used in Ayurvedic medicine, the nutrients in ghee have long been said to cool the body (decrease inflammation), refresh the eyes and enhance vision, fire up the digestion and metabolism, and boost stamina. Ghee is said to sharpen the mind, improving memory, and to protect the body from disease and skin conditions like eczema – plus it's known to increase the luster of the skin and hair, and reduce shadows under the eyes, and has an aphrodisiac effect into the bargain. A bit of a multi-tasker, you might say! While you might instinctively feel that a pure fat like ghee would cause weight gain, quite the opposite appears to be true – by increasing energy levels, it actually helps you to lose weight. It should be consumed in moderation, of course, using a small amount for frying or flavoring a dish.

SKIN-FEEDING NUTRIENTS

- Fatty acids: monounsaturated

- Vitamins:
  A
  D
  E
  K

GINGER

The medicinal and culinary use of ginger goes back centuries and across cultures – there's not really anything else quite like it. As an ingredient, it's used in so many ways around the world – in pickled ginger in Japan, in curries in India and ginger ale in the United States. It's also noted for its medicinal properties, for soothing an upset stomach, for instance, or as part of the classic honey, lemon and ginger combination to help chase away cold and flu symptoms. What is perhaps less well known is that, thanks to its powerful anti-inflammatory nutrients, ginger can do wonders for the complexion, too. Packed with antioxidants, it can help restore radiance by working to reduce inflammation, eliminate acne-causing bacteria and unclog pores, making it a potent addition to the treatment of any serious skin condition, including psoriasis and eczema. The phytochemical gingerol – the spicy constituent of ginger, chemically related to capsaicin in chiles (see p. 143) – works to keep the complexion looking youthful by inhibiting the breakdown of elastin, one of the main causes of wrinkles and fine lines. Boosting blood circulation and cellular turnover, ginger helps to transport nutrients around the system and to eliminate toxins, detoxifying the body, which leads to a happier digestive tract and clearer, more vibrant-looking skin. It also makes a nourishing tea (see p. 259).

SKIN-FEEDING NUTRIENTS

- Dietary fiber
- Minerals:
  copper
  iron
  magnesium
  potassium
- Phytochemicals:
  gingerol
- Vitamins:
  B6 (pyridoxine)
  C

CARROT SOUP (P. 168)

GREEK YOGURT

It can be confusing to navigate the many (often conflicting) nutritional rules in the world of wellness – and Greek yogurt is a good example. Although it's clearly a product made from cow's milk, which can cause skin problems and digestive issues in some people, being a fermented foodstuff means it contains a host of good bacteria – probiotics (literally "pro life") that help to maintain a healthy digestive system, with an additional benefit of keeping the skin clear, too. But not all yogurts are created equal: it's very important to choose full-fat, unsweetened plain Greek yogurt (preferably organic), full of beneficial live bacteria and free from sugar and other additives that can impair their effect in the intestine. A rich source of calcium, Greek yogurt is also a "complete" protein – containing all nine essential amino acids – contributing to the production of new skin cells to ensure a smooth and lustrous complexion. It's interesting to note that Greek yogurt has long been used as a topical treatment to eliminate blemishes and promote radiance. It can be used directly on the face as a mask to soften the skin and calm inflammation, working like a probiotic does in the gut. Indeed, probiotic skincare, based on this principle, is becoming very popular.

SKIN-FEEDING NUTRIENTS

- Minerals:
  calcium
  iodine
  phosphorus
  zinc
- Probiotics
- Protein:
  all nine essential
    amino acids

- Vitamins:
  B2 (riboflavin)
  B6 (pyridoxine)
  B12 (cobalamin)

K ALE

THE DETOX SUPERSTAR

You've probably heard about the countless wonders of kale by now – it's been much lauded as a superfood thanks to its multitude of nutrients and its ability to help the body eliminate waste. In fact, it's one of the most nutrient-dense foods on the planet. It's important to eat dark leafy greens as part of any skin-feeding diet, as they're such a concentrated source of all the things the complexion needs. Absolutely loaded with vitamin K (at about 600 percent of the recommended daily amount per serving), kale helps to strengthen blood vessels, boost the circulation and protect the liver. The anti-inflammatory properties of kale also address bloating – which is good news for the face, as it helps to reduce puffiness as well as redness, making it perfect for treating skin conditions like rosacea. Kale is rich in lutein and zeaxanthin, too, carotenoids that absorb UV light, protecting against free-radical damage and acting like a kind of inner sunscreen. In addition to a wide range and high concentration of vitamins and minerals, kale also contains omega-3 fatty acid, excellent for keeping the complexion supple and nourished from within. Helping to increase the rate of cell turnover and reducing dryness, kale is incredible as part of any radiance-restoring regimen.

SKIN-FEEDING NUTRIENTS

- Dietary fiber
- Fatty acids: omega-3
- Minerals:
  calcium
  copper
  iron
  magnesium
  manganese
  otassium
  phosphorus
  selenium
  zinc

- Phytochemicals: carotenoids (lutein, zeaxanthin)
- Vitamins:
  A
  B1 (thiamine)
  B2 (riboflavin)
  B3 (niacin)
  B6 (pyridoxine)
  B9 (folate)
  choline
  C
  E
  K

KALE SOUP (P. 166)

L EMON

THE NATURAL PURIFIER

I don't know about you, but I couldn't live without lemons – they're such a vital part of my everyday life. I use them for flavoring pretty much everything and often start my day with a glass of lemon, ginger and hot water to kick-start my metabolism and stimulate the liver, helping to flush out any toxins. Lemons are packed with vitamin C, the number-one skin brightener and an essential antioxidant in the production of collagen for youthful-looking skin. Vitamin C is also hugely helpful in treating stress, as it addresses adrenal fatigue, which is brought about by high levels of the stress hormone cortisol. Known for their ability to aid weight loss, lemons have been used for centuries for this purpose – helping the body to rid itself of unwanted waste more efficiently. For me, the biggest selling point of the lemon is its zesty flavor – I naturally associate it with "freshness" and love how eating or drinking anything lemon based makes me feel.

SKIN-FEEDING NUTRIENTS

- Dietary fiber:
  pectin
- Minerals:
  potassium

- Phytochemicals:
  citric acid
  limonoids
- Vitamins:
  C

PINE NUT

THE SKIN-FEEDING SEED

Did you know that pine nuts are not really nuts but seeds? And that they come from a pine cone? Not just any pine cone (in case you're eyeing up the conifers in your garden); the cones/seeds need to be large enough to be worth the fiddly business of harvesting them. A major species for pine nuts is the stone pine, grown in the Mediterranean region for thousands of years for this very purpose. Indeed, pine nuts have been eaten since ancient times for their nutritional benefits and incredible nutty flavor. They also share many of the same nutrients that make nuts so beneficial for our health. In particular, they're known for their ability to keep the heart healthy: the majority of the fat in the seeds is made up of monounsaturated fatty acids, which helps the cardiovascular system to stay strong. It's this type of fat that the Mediterranean diet is so rich in, and known to be one of the best for longevity and general heart health. Pine nuts are also packed with antioxidants, including selenium, lutein and vitamins A, B, C, E and K, which all help to combat the signs of aging by fighting free-radical chain reactions, thus keeping the skin looking young and supple, with good elasticity. The anti-inflammatory properties of pine nuts help to address various skin conditions, including itching, psoriasis, acne and eczema.

SKIN-FEEDING NUTRIENTS

- Fatty acids: monounsaturated omega-6
- Minerals:
  copper
  iron
  magnesium
  manganese
  phosphorus
  potassium
  selenium
  zinc
- Phytochemicals: carotenoids (lutein)
- Protein
- Vitamins:
  A
  B1 (thiamine)
  B3 (niacin)
  C
  E
  K

PINE NUT PESTO WITH SPELT PASTA (P. 156)

PUMPKIN

Is there anything that says "autumn" quite as much as a pumpkin? It's become completely synonymous with the season – bittersweet with the ending of summer but a sign that things are about to get a bit more cozy and festive, with more hearty, warming food choices, too, including the classic pumpkin soup (see page 158). In New York as soon the leaves begin to fall and Halloween is fast approaching, squashes become abundant in the supermarkets and you see artistically carved pumpkins on every stoop. Not something that I grew up with, but great fun all the same. Like all orange fruit and vegetables, pumpkin contains carotenoids – pigments responsible for their vibrant color. Potent antioxidants in their own right, these phytonutrients promote a glowing, healthy complexion and help to reverse UV damage – a good thing at the end of summer. Pumpkins are also packed with a host of vitamins and minerals, including vitamin C, which brightens the skin and promotes collagen production, helping to improve firmness and elasticity. The B vitamins assist with a number of skin functions; helping to oxygenate the skin by widening blood vessels, niacin is particularly useful in the treatment of acne. Meanwhile, the minerals in pumpkin interact to repair and replenish skin cells – just what the skin needs to protect it from the ravages of colder weather.

SKIN-FEEDING NUTRIENTS

- Dietary fiber
- Minerals:
  copper
  iron
  magnesium
  manganese
  potassium
  zinc
- Phytochemicals:
  carotenoids
    (alpha- and
    beta-carotene,
    zeaxanthin)
- Vitamins:
  B2 (riboflavin)
  B3 (niacin)
  B6 (pyridoxine)
  B9 (folate)
  C
  E

THE YOUTH-RESTORING FISH

Sardine

The nutritional benefits of oily fish like sardines are so massive that, when I eat them, each mouthful feels as though it's doing me good. If you imagine all the oils concentrated in the flesh of these fish, those are the very oils that you need for your skin. Loaded with omega-3s, essential fatty acids that have to be obtained from the diet as the body can't produce them itself, sardines are known to help promote collagen production, keeping the skin looking plump, smooth and hydrated. The nutrients in sardines offer a host of other benefits, including improved heart health, enhanced brain function and more stable blood sugar levels. They have been shown to help boost the metabolism and decrease inflammation, as well as minimize sebum production and reduce the congestion that leads to blocked pores – making sardines a bit of a miracle worker for the whole body. Nutrients include selenium, which helps to protect the skin from UV light and to repair damage caused by the sun – just the thing after a long summer. Sardines are also a rich source of vitamin D, essential for healthy bones and teeth and good for mental well-being. This vitamin is otherwise obtainable only from sunlight, making a food source particularly important during the colder months when there is less sun. So if it's dark and chilly outside, tucking into a plate of vitamin D–rich sardines should put a smile back on your face – especially when you think of all those wonderful skin-benefiting omega-3s getting to work!

SKIN-FEEDING NUTRIENTS

- Fatty acids:
  omega-3
- Minerals:
  calcium
  selenium
- Protein:
  all nine essential
    amino acids

- Vitamins:
  B3 (niacin)
  B6 (pyridoxine)
  B12 (cobalamin)
  D

SARDINES ON BUCKWHEAT FLATBREADS (P. 160)

W ALNUT

THE ACNE FIGHTER

It's true that most nuts benefit the skin thanks to the healthy fats and wide range of vitamins and minerals they contain, and walnuts are no exception – as you'll see from the impressive line-up of nutrients listed below. Anti-inflammatory in nature, they are excellent for treating "angry" skin conditions like acne, targeting the infection in the sebaceous glands of the skin. A source of selenium, which helps both to protect the skin from UV exposure and treat existing skin damage, walnuts help to act as an internal sunscreen. Helping, too, to oxygenate your blood and boost the circulation, they are very useful for ensuring a good flow of blood and hence nutrients around the body, which in turn will aid the recovery of inflamed skin. Walnuts are also one of the richest plant sources of omega-3 fatty acids, which are essential for soft and plump skin. Eating a handful of walnuts a day will have you pretty much set for antioxidants, which will work to create a more youthful-looking complexion, so be sure to up your intake for overall well-being and a healthy glow.

SKIN-FEEDING NUTRIENTS

- Dietary fiber
- Fatty acids: omega-3
- Minerals
  calcium
  copper
  iron
  magnesium
  manganese
  phosphorus
  potassium
  selenium
  zinc

- Protein: amino acids (arginine)
- Vitamins:
  B1 (thiamine)
  B2 (riboflavin)
  B3 (niacin)
  B5 (pantothenic acid)
  B6 (pyridoxine)
  B9 (folate)
  E
  K

NO-COOK WALNUT BROWNIES (P. 184)

Green protein smoothie

SERVES 2

————

151 CALORIES PER SERVING
(WITHOUT TOPPINGS)

————

- 2 kale leaves, thick
  stems removed
- Small handful of spinach
- Flesh of 1 small avocado,
  chopped
- ½ cup coconut water
- ¾ cup unsweetened almond milk
- 1 date, pitted and chopped

I drink a lot of coconut water, and it's great to have first thing, as it will flush away any toxins. Every ingredient in this recipe has skin-benefiting properties – indeed, each has its own section in this book! Loaded with healthy fats that help to plump and smooth skin as well as vitamin E to help protect it from free-radical damage, this is tailor-made for that early-morning boost – both for energy levels and the overall beauty of the skin.

1. Place all the ingredients in a blender or food processor and whizz until smooth.

Pine nut pesto with spelt pasta

SERVES 2

————

540 CALORIES
PER SERVING

————

- 5 oz spelt pasta
- 3 handfuls of raw pine nuts
- Handful of arugula
- 3 handfuls of fresh basil
- Handful of fresh parsley
- 1 garlic clove
- Juice of ½ lemon
- 1 tbsp extra-virgin olive oil,
  plus extra for drizzling
- 2 oz Parmesan cheese, grated,
  plus extra to serve
- Sea salt and black pepper

Everyone loves pesto, and this is my version – full of flavor and so simple to make. I've paired it with wheat-free pasta for a quick and tasty meal, but it would be great as a side dish to serve with fish or chicken for an added bit of flavor and skin-friendly nutrition. Spelt or brown rice pasta is worth bearing in mind for its low glycemic load (GL). Complex carbs help to moderate the release of insulin, which is good for the skin as continual spikes in insulin from high-GL foods such as sugar may damage collagen and accelerate wrinkles.

1. Cook the pasta in boiling water according to the package instructions (making sure the water is quite salty), then drain.
2. Place all the remaining ingredients in a food processor and blend until the desired consistency is reached, seasoning to taste with salt and pepper.
3. Stir the pesto through the cooked pasta and serve with extra Parmesan and olive oil sprinkled over and some freshly cracked black pepper.

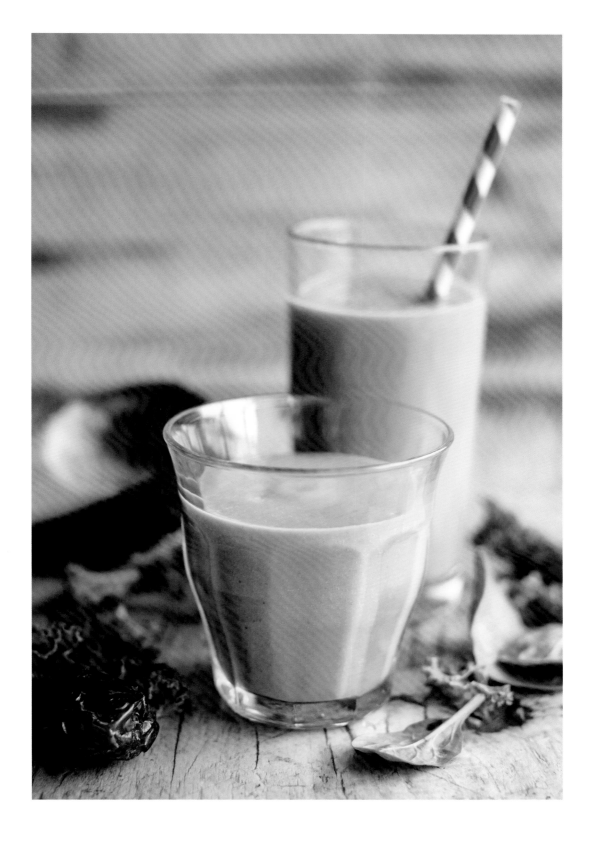

GREEN PROTEIN SMOOTHIE

Roast pumpkin soup

SERVES 4

———

224 CALORIES
PER SERVING

———

- Flesh of 1 small pumpkin, cut into 2-inch chunks (see tip below)
- 1 tbsp olive oil
- 2 tbsp raw coconut oil
- 2 garlic cloves, finely chopped
- 1 shallot, finely chopped
- 5 cups chicken stock (to make your own, see p. 228) or vegetable stock
- Sea salt and black pepper
- Small handful of fresh sage leaves, chopped, to garnish

Sometimes there's no point in fighting tradition: pumpkin soup is as obvious as can be for autumn, but who cares when it's so tasty – and so good for you, too. In my opinion, the pumpkin really has to be roasted first to enhance the sweetness of the flesh and improve the texture. This recipe is creamy without any added dairy and sweet without any sugar. Delicious!

1. Preheat the oven to 425°F.
2. Place the pumpkin in a baking sheet or roasting pan, add the olive oil and a pinch of salt and toss together. Roast in the oven for 30 minutes or until tender.
3. Melt the coconut oil in a large saucepan over medium heat. Add the garlic and shallot and cook for 5 minutes or until the shallot is translucent.
4. Add the roasted pumpkin and the stock to the saucepan and bring to a boil. Reduce the heat and simmer for 20 minutes or until tender. Check for seasoning, adding salt and pepper to taste.
5. Blend the soup until smooth in a food processor, or in the pan using an immersion blender, and garnish with the chopped sage before serving.

TIP

- Be sure to reserve a handful of the pumpkin seeds and cook them in the oven at the same time. Scatter them in a separate large pan and cook for about 5 minutes, keeping an eye on them and turning frequently to ensure they don't burn. They're highly nutritious in their own right and an excellent source of roughage – the roasted seeds can be sprinkled over the finished soup.

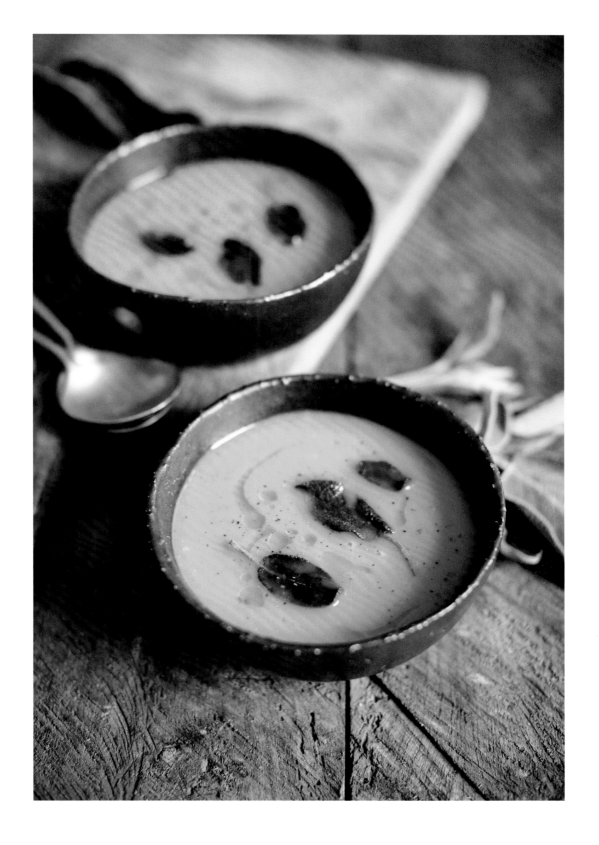

Sardines on buckwheat flatbreads

SERVES 4

———

280 CALORIES
PER SERVING

———

- 4 tbsp buckwheat flour, plus extra for dusting
- Raw coconut oil, for frying
- 4 fresh sardines, gutted and cleaned (ask your fishmonger to do this)
- Handful of fresh parsley, finely chopped, plus extra to serve
- Juice of ½ lemon
- Salt and freshly ground black pepper

TO SERVE
- 1 watermelon radish (or a handful of red radishes), sliced into thin circles
- Lemon wedges

I keep cans of sardines in my pantry to have as a simple snack – great on toast with a sprinkling of sea salt and cracked black pepper. While they're lower in mercury than other sea fish, it's important to buy wild-caught sardines and opt for those packed in water or oil, rather than brine – you can always add the salt later. Even better, buy them fresh from your fishmonger. Bursting with flavor, they need very little to enhance them – just a few herbs and a squeeze of lemon.

1. Place the flour in a bowl with 2 tablespoons of water and knead together to make a dough. (Buckwheat can be quite sticky so you may need to add more flour.)
2. Roll the dough into a tube and slice into four sections. On a work surface lightly dusted with flour, roll each piece out into a flatbread about ⅛ inch thick.
3. Heat a little coconut oil in a medium nonstick skillet over medium heat, add a flatbread and cook on each side for 2–3 minutes or until browned. Transfer to a plate and cook the remaining flatbreads in the same way.
4. Meanwhile, cook the sardines. Melt 1 tablespoon of coconut oil in a large skillet and add the sardines, parsley and lemon juice. Season with a little salt and pepper and cook over medium heat for 5 minutes on each side or until cooked through (see tip).
5. To assemble, place slices of radish on top of each flatbread, top with a sardine and serve with extra parsley sprinkled over and a wedge of lemon.

TIP
- The only downside of cooking fresh sardines is that they will stink up your house! To avoid this, cook them outdoors on the grill.

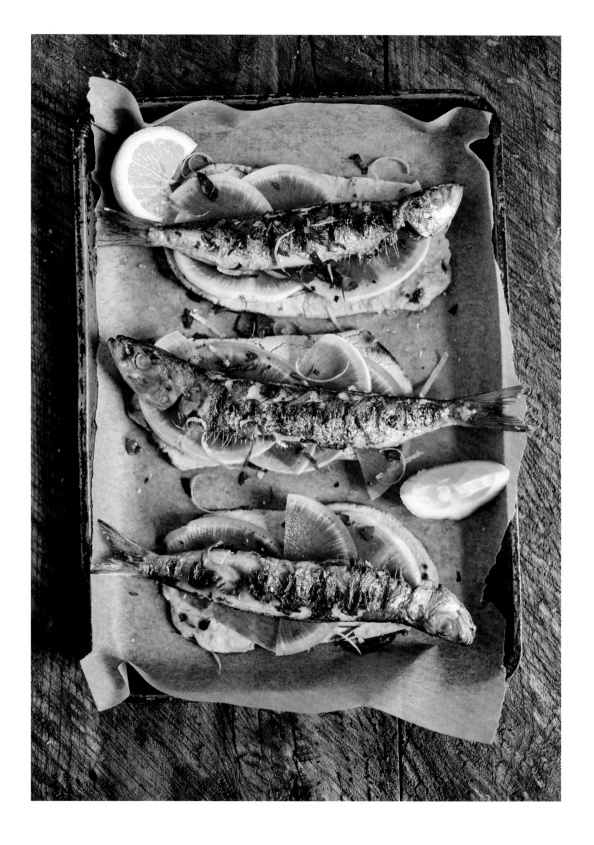

Chickpea and chicken tagine

SERVES 2

———

415 CALORIES
PER SERVING

———

- 4 skinless and boneless
  chicken thighs, diced
- 1 medium onion, chopped
- 1 cinnamon stick
- A few strands of saffron
- 1 cup canned chickpeas,
  drained and rinsed
- 1 large yellow pepper
- 1 large red pepper
- 1 tbsp olive oil
- 4 dried apricots, chopped
- Small handful of fresh
  flat-leaf parsley, chopped
- Juice of 1–2 lemons
- Sea salt and black pepper

Chickpeas are a great, inexpensive alternative to traditional carbs. All the flavors and textures meld together, offset by the spices and the sweetness of the dried fruits.

1. Add the chicken pieces to a large saucepan with the onion, cinnamon stick, saffron and chickpeas.
2. Pour in water to cover by 1 inch, then bring to a boil. Once boiling, cover the pan with a lid and reduce the heat. Leave to simmer gently for 1 hour.
3. Meanwhile, preheat the oven to 400°F.
4. Place the peppers on a baking sheet, drizzle with oil and roast in the oven for about 25 minutes or until tender.
5. Once cooked, cut the peppers into small pieces, removing the stalks and seeds.
6. When it has been simmering for 1 hour, stir in the peppers and the apricots. Cook for 40 minutes.
7. Season to taste, then sprinkle with parsley, squeeze over the lemon juice and serve immediately.

Tzatziki

SERVES 2
AS A SIDE DISH

———

57 CALORIES
PER SERVING

———

- 2 tbsp natural Greek yogurt
- ½ cucumber, finely chopped
- 6 sprigs of mint, finely chopped
- 1 tbsp apple cider vinegar
  or mint sauce

There's nothing quite like a bowl of homemade tzatziki as a side dish to freshen the palate – especially with spicy food like curry – or to enjoy as a dip with gluten-free seeded crackers. Full of fresh flavor, this recipe has a host of skin benefits, the cucumber and mint being excellent skin-feeding ingredients in their own right.

1. Place the yogurt in a small bowl with the cucumber and mint.
2. Add the apple cider vinegar or mint sauce and stir everything together.

BREAKFAST SKIN BOOSTER

Try eating a bowl of Greek yogurt, blueberries (see p. 37) and manuka honey for breakfast for a week. It will help address acne and decrease inflammation.

CHICKPEA (P. 142)   GREEK YOGURT (P. 149)

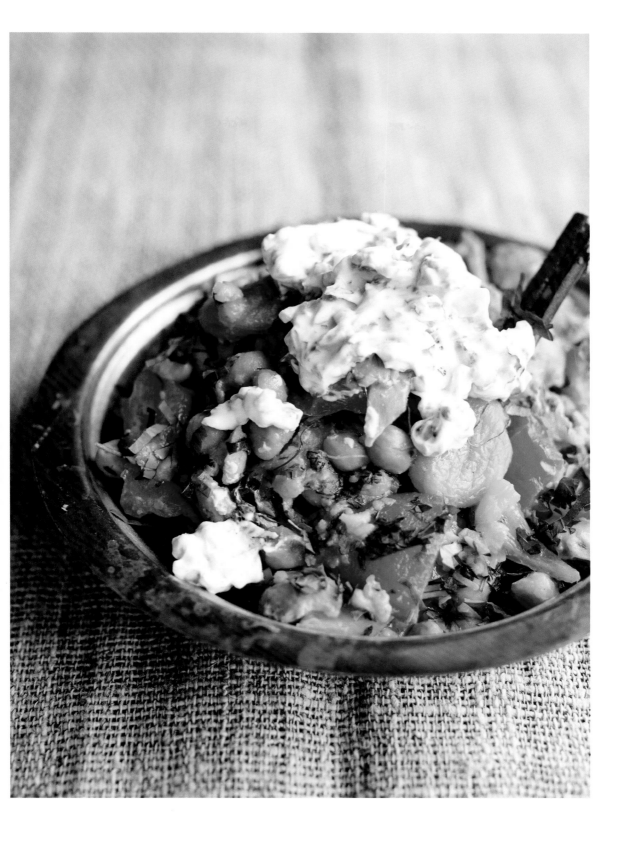

CHICKPEA AND CHICKEN TAGINE WITH TZATZIKI

Chicken satay

SERVES 2

————

449 CALORIES
PER SERVING

————

FOR THE CHICKEN SKEWERS
- 10 oz skinless chicken breasts, sliced into strips
- ½ cup coconut milk
- 1 tbsp honey
- 1–2 tbsp soy sauce
- Handful of fresh cilantro, finely chopped
- 3 garlic cloves, finely diced
- Pinch of ground turmeric
- 1 tsp ground cumin
- 1 fresh red chile, seeded and finely chopped

FOR THE SATAY SAUCE
- Handful of raw peanuts, crushed
- 1 tbsp soy sauce
- 1–2 tsp ground turmeric
- 1 tsp palm sugar or honey
- 1 tbsp coconut milk
- Handful of fresh cilantro, finely chopped

There are too many ways of cooking chicken to mention here, and you'll see that chicken is included in quite a few recipes in this book, from the Chickpea and Chicken Tagine in this section to my Classic Roast Chicken (see pp. 162 and 230). I love this chicken satay dish; as well as reminding me of trips to Thailand, it helps fill me up, and is super tasty and amazing for the health of my skin. Let's face it, everyone likes satay chicken. You can throw this in the oven or on the barbecue, or even cook in foil.

1. If using wooden skewers (you'll need about six), soak them in water for 20 minutes before using.
2. Place all the ingredients for the chicken skewers in a large bowl and combine well, massaging the marinade ingredients into the meat. If you have time, leave the chicken to marinate for about 2 hours in the fridge.
3. Preheat the oven to 400°F.
4. Transfer the marinated chicken to a baking sheet and bake in the oven for 15–20 minutes, turning them halfway through, or until cooked (see tip below).
5. Meanwhile, make the satay sauce. Place all the ingredients in a bowl, add a tablespoon of water and blend using an immersion blender.
6. Thread the cooked chicken strips on to the skewers and serve with the satay sauce, either poured over the chicken or in a bowl for dipping.

TIPS
- If you like, you can cook the chicken pieces in a skillet on the burner or on the barbecue for 10–15 minutes or until cooked through and slightly charred.
- Try using shrimp instead of chicken.

CHICKEN (P. 141)

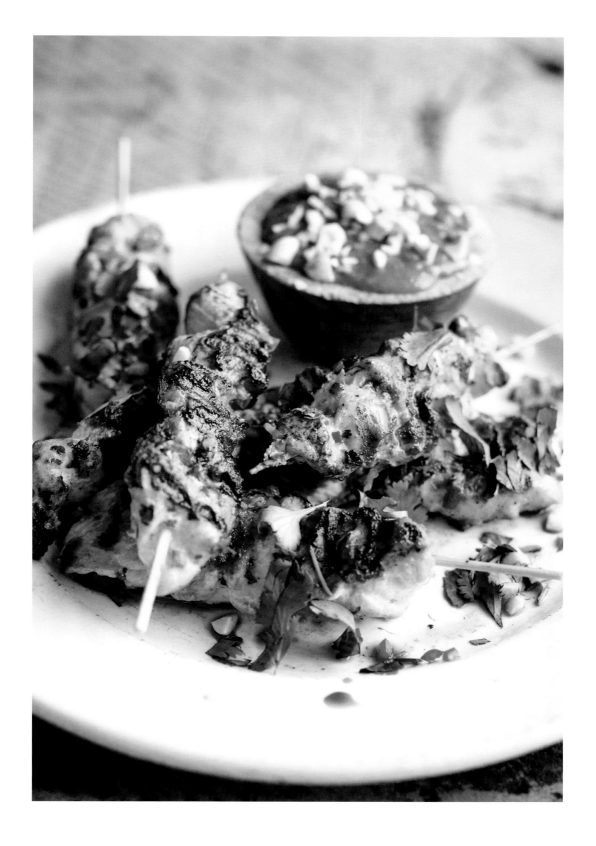

Kale soup

SERVES 2

———

185 CALORIES
PER SERVING

———

- 1 large fennel bulb,
  roughly chopped
- 1 leek, roughly chopped
- 1 tbsp olive oil
- 1 tbsp raw coconut oil
- 1 onion, chopped
- 2 garlic cloves, finely
  chopped
- 1 tbsp vegetable bouillon
  powder or 1 vegetable
  stock cube
- 10 kale leaves, large stems
  removed, roughly chopped
- Handful of spinach
- Sea salt and black pepper
- 1 tsp grated nutmeg,
  to serve

I'm not a huge fan of strict "detox" diets, but I do know when it's time to rein in any bad behavior or over-consumption and "eat clean" – and this soup really helps me to do that. I always make it during such times and the nutrient boost really helps me to feel like I'm back on track; it tastes amazing and filling and works to flush out the system, all the while feeding my skin and restoring a glow. This is a really easy meal.

1.   Preheat the oven to 400°F.
2.   Place the fennel and leek on a baking sheet or roasting pan, add the olive oil and toss together. Bake in the oven for 15–20 minutes.
3.   Melt the coconut oil in a large saucepan over low heat. Add the onion and garlic, place a lid on the pan and sweat for about 5 minutes or until the onion is translucent and softened.
4.   Pour 5 cups of water into the pan and add the vegetable bouillon powder or stock cube. Add the roasted fennel and the leek, along with half the chopped-up kale leaves. Season with salt and pepper and give everything a stir.
5.   Bring to a boil and leave to bubble away for 20 minutes. Add the remaining kale and all the spinach, then simmer over medium-low heat for another 10 minutes.
6.   Let cool down slightly, then purée until smooth in a stand-alone blender or using an immersion blender. Reheat as needed and sprinkle with nutmeg to serve.

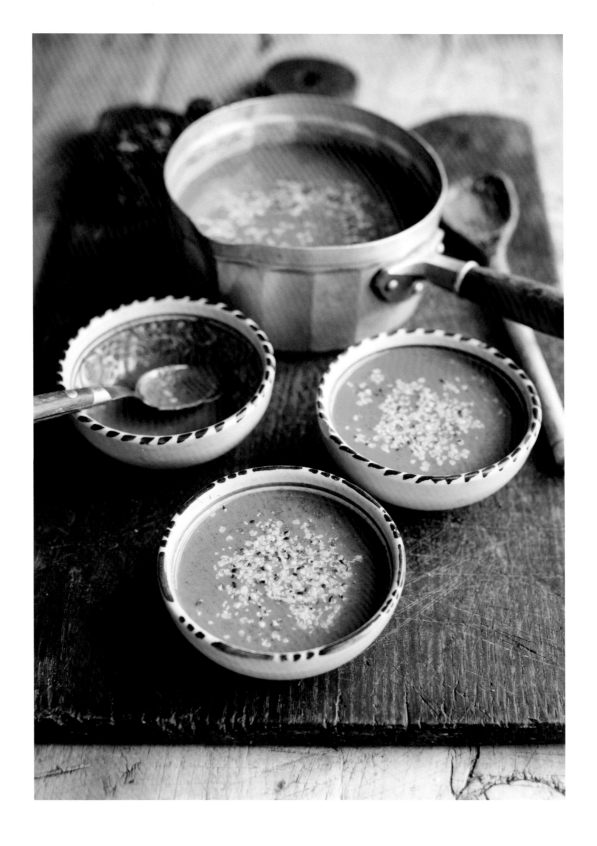

Roasted garlic spread

MAKES 1 ROASTED
GARLIC BULB

————

12 CALORIES
PER CLOVE

————

- 1 large whole garlic bulb
- 1 tbsp olive oil

This recipe for roasted garlic is just so simple – but that's the beauty of it. I like to use the garlic paste from the roasted bulbs as an alternative to butter or to add to other dishes. I simply squeeze the roasted garlic from the cloves to add to my dish as I'm cooking. Cooked like this, garlic tastes very sweet and is not so strong-smelling. (Though I love garlic, as a makeup artist I'm all too aware of the danger of getting raw garlic on my fingers, so I try not to cook it before I go to work!) Garlic is incredible for skin and your health in general – a little nutritional miracle.

1. Preheat the oven to 400°F.
2. Cut the top off the garlic bulb so that the cloves are revealed, then drizzle with oil. Wrap it in foil, place on baking sheet and bake for 40 minutes. Remove from the oven and leave to cool.
3. Once cooled, the roasted garlic bulb can be kept in the fridge to use as needed. Simply scoop out the roasted flesh from the individual cloves using a knife, or just squeeze the flesh from the cloves and use as a butter.

Carrot soup

SERVES 2
AS A SIDE DISH

————

89 CALORIES
PER SERVING

————

- 1 medium onion, chopped
- 3 large carrots, chopped
- 1 garlic clove, crushed
- ½-inch knob of fresh ginger, peeled and finely chopped
- Pinch of ground cumin
- Sea salt and black pepper
- Handful of fresh parsley

I love to make this soup in the autumn – the colors are so right for the season, while the peppery flavor of the ginger is both warming and refreshing, helping to keep my digestion fired up and my skin looking clear and supple.

1. Fill a large saucepan with 5 cups of water, add the onion, carrots, garlic, ginger and cumin and bring to a boil.
2. Reduce the heat and simmer for about 15 minutes or until the carrots are soft.
3. Blend the soup until smooth in a food processor or using an immersion blender. Season to taste with salt and pepper and top with the parsley to serve.

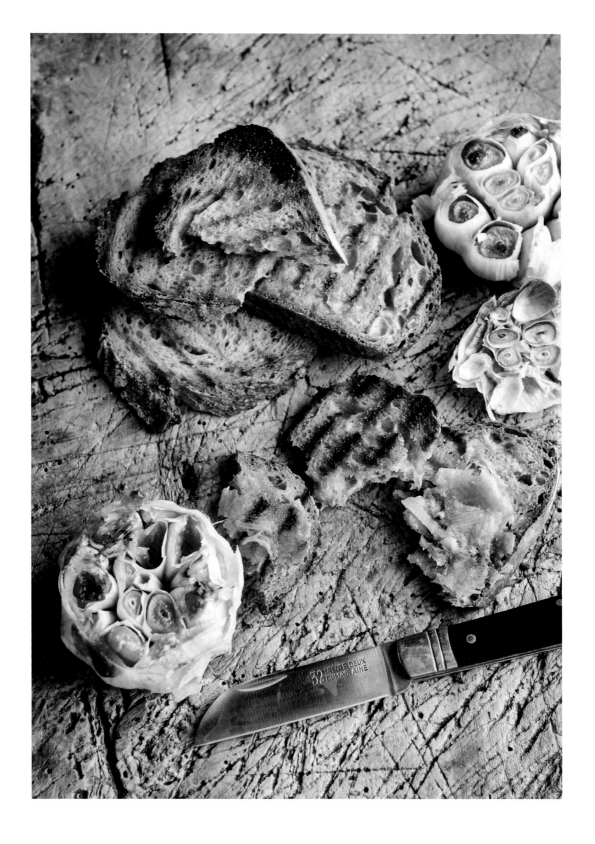

ROASTED GARLIC SPREAD

Sticky chile beef

SERVES 2

————

250 CALORIES
PER SERVING

————

FOR THE MARINADE
- 1 fresh red chile, seeded and finely chopped
- ½-inch knob of fresh ginger, peeled and grated
- 1 garlic clove, finely chopped
- 1 shallot, finely chopped
- 1 tbsp honey
- Small handful of fresh cilantro, finely chopped
- Juice of ½ lime
- 1 tsp finely chopped lemongrass
- 2 tbsp soy sauce

- 6 thin beef steaks (minute steaks), cut into thin little strips
- 1 tsp raw coconut oil

TO SERVE (OPTIONAL)
- Radish Salad (p. 58)

When the weather turns a bit miserable, it makes sense to eat a warming, protein-based dish like this one. It's super quick to make and easy to digest, and wakes up the senses with its delicious flavors. I was inspired to make it after tasting the amazing spicy stir-fries in Thailand. I've used beef in this recipe – another food that's great for your skin – but you can substitute with chicken or fish, if you prefer. My friends love this dish!

1. Place all the marinade ingredients in a bowl and mix together well.
2. Add the beef and leave to marinate for 1–2 hours (the longer the better, though you can cook the beef right away if you're pushed for time).
3. Melt the coconut oil in a large skillet over high heat. Add the marinated beef and stir-fry for about 5 minutes until it becomes sticky and very browned.
4. Serve with Radish Salad if you like.

CRUSHED RED PEPPER FLAKES
A really easy way to add chile to dishes is in the form of dried crushed red pepper flakes, which you can add to anything, anywhere. They're not expensive and have all the circulation-boosting benefits of fresh chiles.

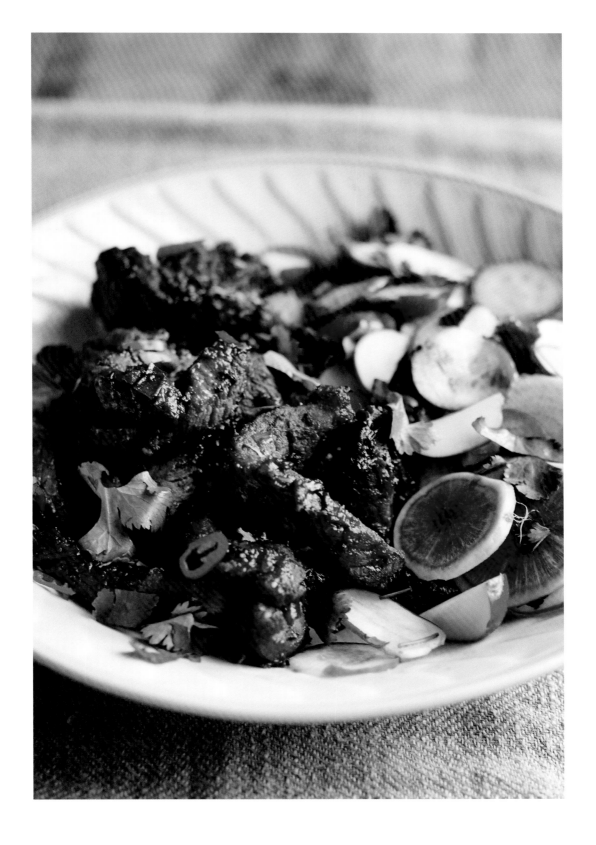

Brown rice and vegetable pilaf

SERVES 6-8

————

398 CALORIES
PER SERVING

————

- ¼ cup coconut milk
- 1 shallot, finely chopped
- 2 garlic cloves, finely chopped
- 1 tbsp grated fresh root ginger
- Flesh of 1–4 pumpkin or butternut squash, diced
- 1 eggplant, diced
- 1 piece of tenderstem broccoli, diced
- Handful of green beans, cut into short lengths
- Handful of spinach
- 1 tbsp curry powder
- 1–4 tsp ground turmeric
- ¾ cup brown jasmine rice
- 3 tbsp soy sauce
- 1 tbsp miso paste
- 1 cinnamon stick
- 4 cardamom pods
- 1 bay leaf
- Sea salt and black pepper

Brown rice is so tasty that I'll often eat it on its own or with some tamari and a bit of broccoli chucked in with it. It's also great with other dishes, of course. I love cooking spicy dishes when the weather starts to turn, serving them with brown rice – they're so satisfying, keeping you full for hours. I adore Indian food but sometimes it can be a bit greasy when it doesn't have to be. The recipe I've included here is low in fat but still high in flavor and with other skin-feeding ingredients, such as eggplant, spinach and garlic. It would team well with a bowl of Tzatziki or Cucumber and Mango Salsa (see pp. 162 and 126).

1. Heat the coconut milk in a large saucepan. Add the shallot, garlic and ginger and simmer over low heat for 5 minutes.
2. Add the pumpkin and eggplant and cook for another 5 minutes, then add the broccoli, beans and spinach and cook for another 5 minutes, adding a splash of water if needed, until all the vegetables have softened.
3. Add the curry powder and turmeric, and stir in well, seasoning to taste with salt and pepper.
4. Add the rice and add the soy sauce and miso paste, stirring in to combine. Pour in 1 cup water and stir well, then add the cinnamon stick, cardamom and bay leaf.
5. Cover the pan with a lid and bring to a boil, then reduce the heat and simmer for 30–35 minutes or until the rice is cooked.
6. Remove from the heat and leave for 10 minutes with the lid on. Discard the cardamom pods, bay leaf and cinnamon stick before serving.

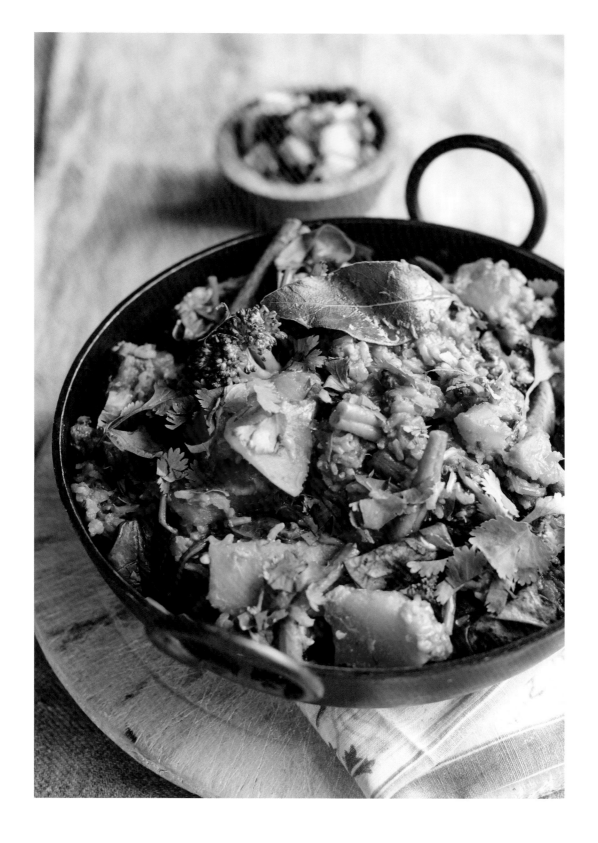

Meatballs
arrabbiata

SERVES 4

————

652 CALORIES
PER SERVING

————

FOR THE MEATBALLS
- 1 lb ground beef
- Handful of fresh parsley, finely chopped
- 1 tsp butter or coconut oil
- Sea salt and black pepper
- Small handful of fresh basil, torn

FOR THE
ARRABBIATA SAUCE
- 1 onion, finely chopped
- 2 garlic cloves, finely chopped
- 1 fresh red chile, seeded and finely chopped
- 14½-oz can of tomatoes

I don't eat a lot of meat and when I do I normally choose chicken or fish – red meat is not my usual thing. Having said that, I recognize that a lot of people do like meat. I also realize that when my body feels like it is running on empty it is often because of a lack of iron. This meatball recipe feels hearty, tastes delicious – and you know it's working to improve your complexion and health as you eat it, too. Great served with pasta or brown rice (see p. 140).

1. Preheat the oven to 400°F.
2. Place the ground beef and parsley in a bowl and season with salt and pepper. Use your hands to mix the ingredients together, then divide the mixture into eight sections and roll each piece into a ball.
3. Melt the butter or coconut oil in a large skillet over medium-high heat. Add the meatballs and sear on all sides to brown them, then transfer to a medium ovenproof dish and bake in the oven for 15 minutes.
4. While the meatballs are cooking, make the arrabbiata sauce. Add the onion, garlic and chile to the skillet and cook over medium heat for about 5 minutes or until the onion is softened and translucent.
5. Add the tomatoes to the pan, then bring to a simmer and cook for 5 minutes. Season to taste with salt and pepper.
6. Remove the meatballs from the oven and pour over the sauce, scattering with fresh basil to serve.

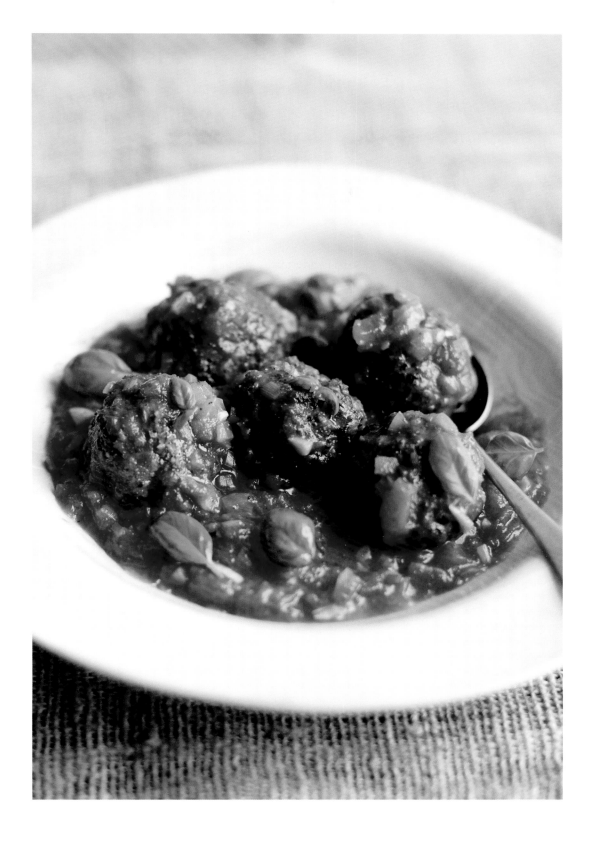

Paleo roti

MAKES 6—8 ROTIS

————

80 CALORIES
PER ROTI

————

- 1 cup golden flaxseed meal
- 1 cup tapioca flour
- 1¼ cups coconut milk
- Pinch of sea salt
- 1 tbsp ghee

This recipe harks back to a Ghanaian dish that my friend Vanessa's mum used to make and which I loved. When I went to their home, I'd always ask: "Has your mum made any rotis?" Her name is Yvonne and she was, and is, a great cook. (When she reads this, she'll probably tell me off for not having been around to see her in ages.) Fried in ghee, the rotis are made with flaxseed – a source of phytoestrogens that work in the body in a similar way to estrogen. A diet rich in phytoestrogens is said to help with hormone imbalances that may affect the condition of your skin.

1. Heat a medium nonstick skillet, at least 9 inches in diameter, over medium heat.
2. Mix all the ingredients together in a jar or bowl, and pour half the batter into the pan, spreading it out with a spoon so that it covers the bottom of the pan.
3. After 2–3 minutes, or once the batter fluffs up and looks firm/mostly cooked, flip it over with a spatula to cook the other side. (Be patient, as this takes time. If you are worried about the outside burning, just lower the heat.) Transfer the cooked roti to a plate.
4. Pour the remaining batter into the pan and cook both sides as above. (See tips below.)

TIPS
- You will notice that as the batter sits in your jar or bowl, it will become thicker. That's because flaxseed meal soaks up moisture quickly. Feel free to thin out the batter by adding more coconut milk. You don't have to do this, but if you don't, just bear in mind that your second roti might be thicker than the first.
- If the middle of the rotis still seem slightly undercooked, place them on a baking sheet and cook in the oven at 400°F for 10–15 minutes.

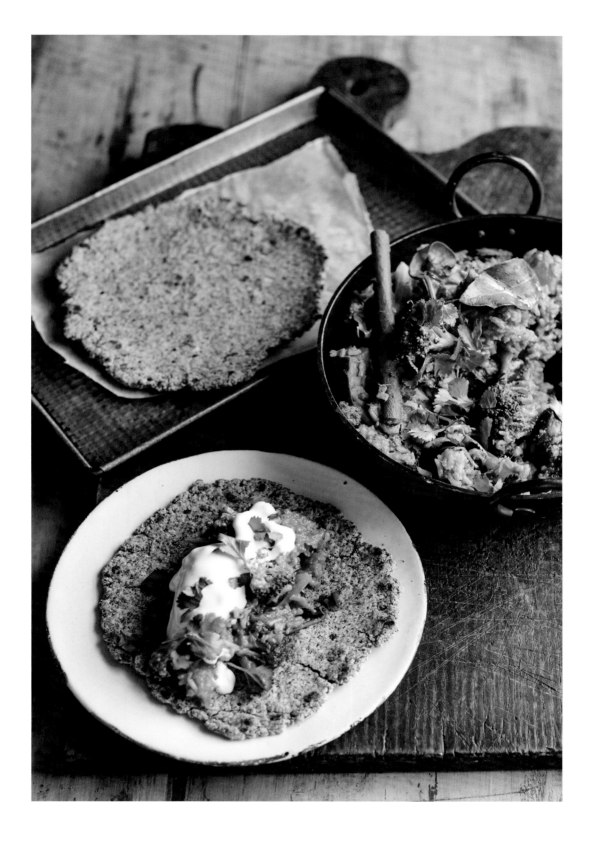

PALEO ROTI WITH BROWN RICE AND VEGETABLE PILAF (P. 172)

Date
energy bites

MAKES 10 BALLS

————

160 CALORIES
PER BALL

————

- 4 oz pitted dates
- 4 oz dried apple rings
- ½ cup unsalted
  dry-roasted almonds
- ½ cup gluten-free
  rolled oats
- 1 tbsp maple syrup
- 1 tsp ground cinnamon
- Handful of pistachios,
  finely chopped

These date bites are great when I have an early call time and don't feel like eating breakfast right away; they give me the quick hit of energy I need.

1. Cover the dates in hot water and leave to soak for 10 minutes to soften. Drain and squeeze out any water.
2. Place in a food processor with all the the remaining ingredients except the pistachios, add 1 tablespoon of water and blend until the mixture turns into a paste with a sticky, dough-like consistency. Add another tablespoon of water to loosen further, if needed.
3. Scoop out tablespoons of the mixture and, between clean, wet hands, roll into ten balls. Place the pistachios into a bowl and roll each ball in the nuts to coat.
4. Store in an airtight container in the fridge or freezer.

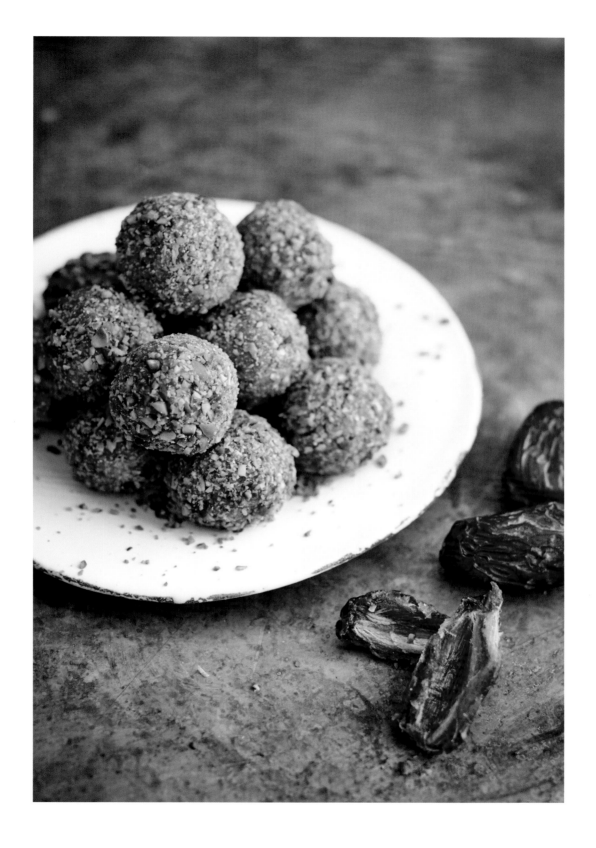

Stewed apples
with cinnamon

SERVES 2

———

238 CALORIES
PER SERVING

———

- 6 cooking apples, peeled, cored and cut into bite-sized pieces
- 1 cup boiling water
- 1 tbsp honey, plus extra to serve
- 1½ tsp vanilla extract
- 1 tsp ground cinnamon
- 2 tbsp natural Greek yogurt, to serve (optional)

My mum would make a whole array of different dishes using stewed apples. It tastes quite naughty, but with only a spoonful of honey to sweeten it, there's nothing but the healthy deliciousness of the stewed apple.

1. Place the apple pieces in a medium saucepan and add the hot water. Add the honey, vanilla and cinnamon and stir to combine.
2. Cover, bring to a simmer and cook over gentle heat for 20 minutes or so.
3. When the apples are soft and caramel colored, remove from the heat and serve with the yogurt (if using) and additional honey.

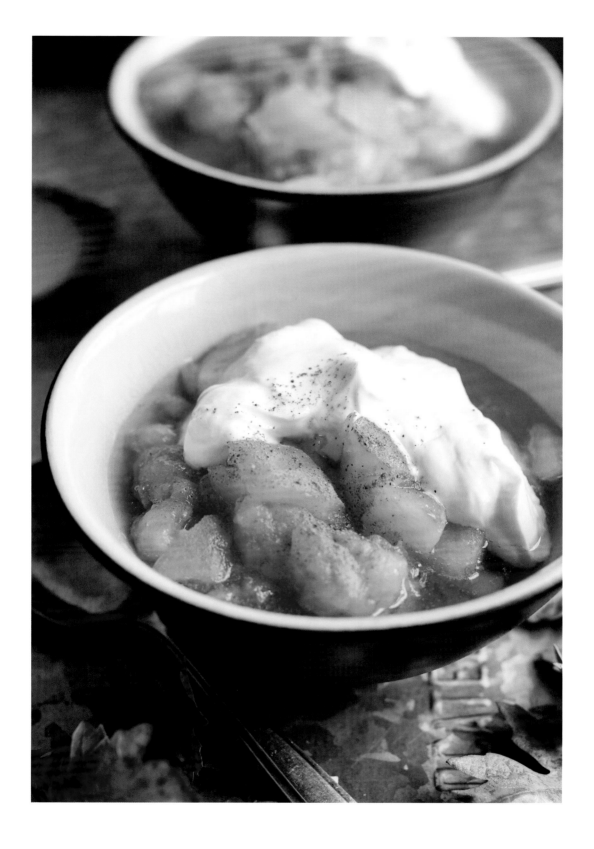

Mini
lemon tarts

MAKES 12 TARTS

———

214 CALORIES
PER SERVING

———

FOR THE CRUST
- 6 tbsp coconut oil, melted, plus extra for greasing
- ¾ cup blanched almond flour, plus extra for dusting
- 3 tbsp palm sugar

FOR THE LEMON CURD
- 4 large egg yolks
- 2 tbsp maple syrup
- 1 tsp grated lemon zest
- 6 tbsp fresh lemon juice
- 6 tbsp coconut oil, melted

A lemon-based dessert after a meal is so refreshing, I always think, helping to cleanse the palate. The coconut oil used here contains medium-chain fatty acids that are quickly converted to energy, speeding up the metabolism and improving digestion, with benefits for the skin. The flavor of coconut imparts a natural sweetness, which is useful to bear in mind if you're trying to cut back on sugar in your diet. That said, these little tarts do contain some sugar, so are best reserved for a special treat!

1. Preheat the oven to 425°F and grease the molds of a 12-cup mini muffin tin with coconut oil.
2. Place the ingredients for the tart crust in a bowl and mix to form a dough. Transfer to a work surface lightly dusted with flour and roll out to about 1 inch thick. Use an 3-inch cutter to stamp out 12 pastry circles.
3. Press the pastry circles into the molds of the tin and bake for 8–10 minutes or until golden. Make sure you keep an eye on them as they can quickly burn.
4. Remove from the oven and reduce the heat to 400°F.
5. Meanwhile, make the lemon curd. Place the egg yolks, maple syrup, lemon zest and lemon juice in a medium heatproof bowl and set over a medium saucepan of gently simmering water. Whisk the mixture constantly for 7–10 minutes or until the curd thickens, then remove from the heat and mix in the coconut oil.
6. Fill each crust with lemon curd and bake in the oven for 8–10 minutes or until golden.
7. Once baked, leave to cool down fully in the muffin tin and chill in the fridge for 15 minutes before removing from the tin. Keep stored in the fridge for up to 5 days.

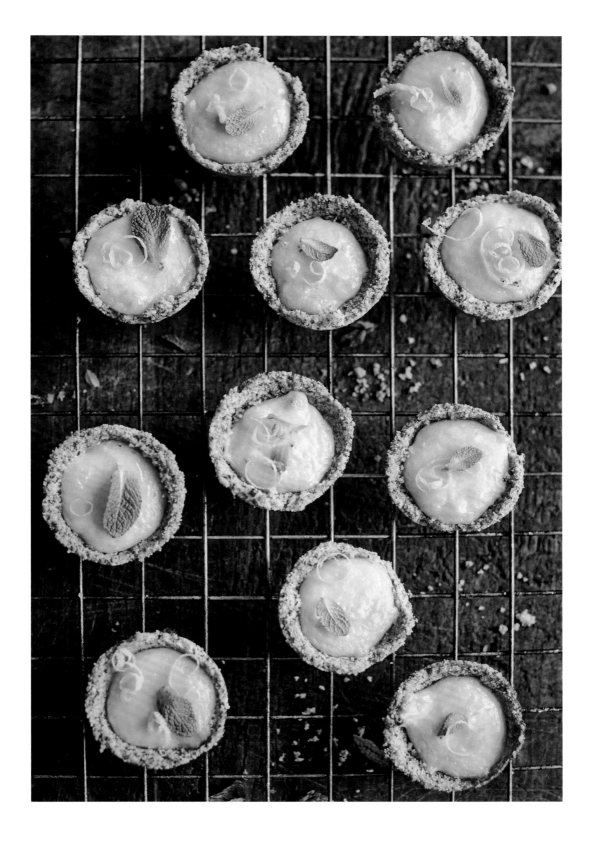

No-cook
walnut brownies

MAKES 16 BROWNIES

————

180 CALORIES
PER BROWNIE

————

- 5 oz pitted dates
- 10 oz raw walnut pieces
- ¼ cup raw cacao
  (or cocoa) powder
- 2 tsp vanilla extract

Walnuts should really be combined with something that has a lot of water in it – such as a salad – so including this recipe is a bit of a cheat. On the other hand, these brownies are outrageously delicious, plus they contain no gluten or refined sugars – just skin-friendly dates for a touch of natural sweetness – and they need no baking. Take them with you to work as a snack, or invite some friends over to enjoy them – they'll be clamoring for the recipe!

1. Cover the dates in warm water and leave to soak for 10 minutes to soften.
2. In a food processor, blend the walnuts and cacao powder until the nuts are finely ground.
3. Drain the soaked dates, squeeze out any excess water and add to the food processor with the vanilla extract. Process until the mixture sticks together and forms a ball, adding up to 2 tablespoons of water, if desired, for moister brownies.
4. Line an 8-inch square baking pan with parchment paper and press the brownie mixture into the pan.
5. Cover the pan with plastic wrap and place in the fridge to chill for at least 2 hours or until set. Cut the mixture into 16 squares to serve.
6. The brownies can be kept in an airtight container in the fridge for up to 5 days or frozen for up to 2 weeks.

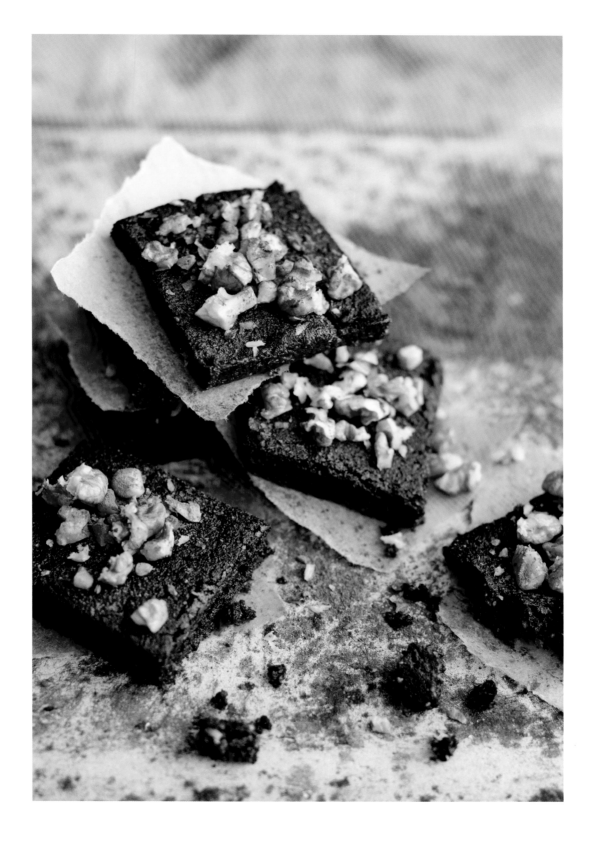

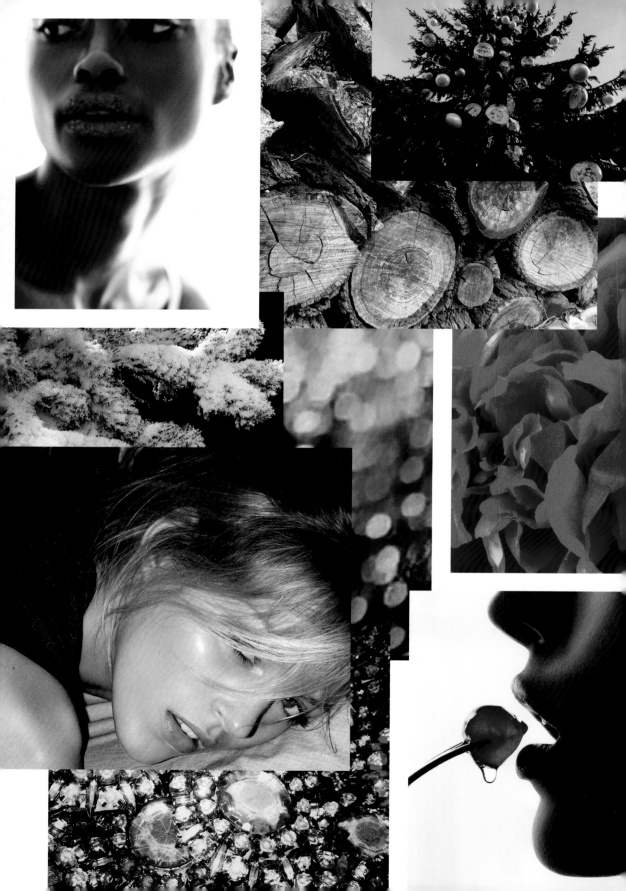

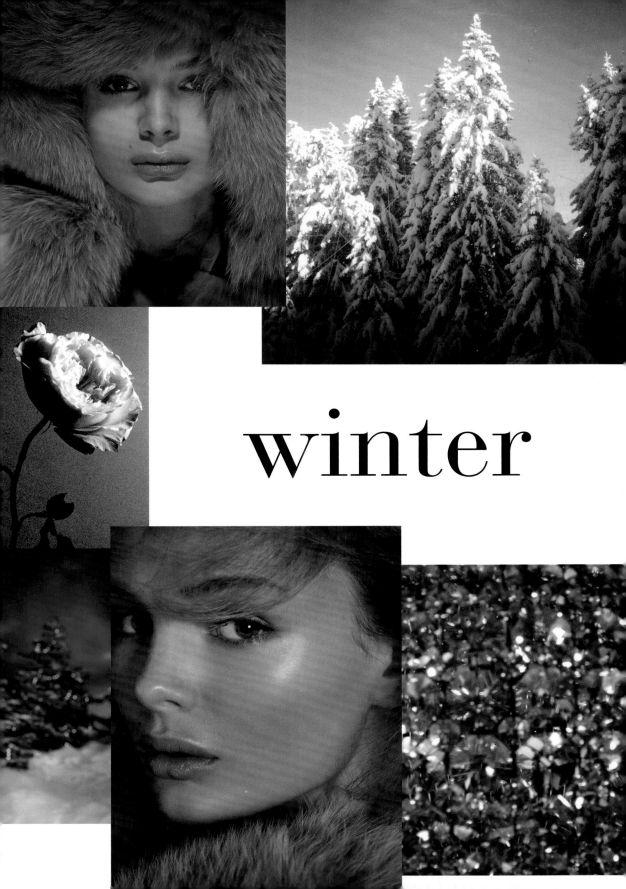

winter

The cold war

This is hibernation time, dashing back from work to get into the heat, or scuttling from home to taxi to a party. But you should try to be outdoors for at least 20 minutes each day, both for the fresh air and vitamin D. I know it's hard, but it will help stave off cold bugs and keep the winter blues away.

When it gets really cold – as it can do in New York – I turn into a wildling from *Game of Thrones*, complete with hat or hood, good gloves, boots and wrapped up in multiple layers.

Winter can be hard going for the skin. Freezing winds and cold temperatures take their toll, but we also spend more time indoors, exposed to almost constant heating, which dries the skin out, causing tightness, itchiness and irritation. Richer products will help keep the skin nourished. Dry brushing before a shower or a bath is always good, both to remove any dry skin and to get the circulation going. It's tempting to have a really hot bath, but this is best avoided, as extreme heat can cause broken veins.

Drinking plenty of water is important – it's essential for hydration and to replenish the blood in its vital role of carrying nutrients and oxygen around the body. A glass of hot water and lemon can be a great way to start the day: it kick-starts the metabolism and rehydrates. I make sure my food is full of essential fatty acids, antioxidants and good oils and I eat lots of fish, sesame seeds and tofu, which are rich in omega-3 and improve the skin's suppleness.

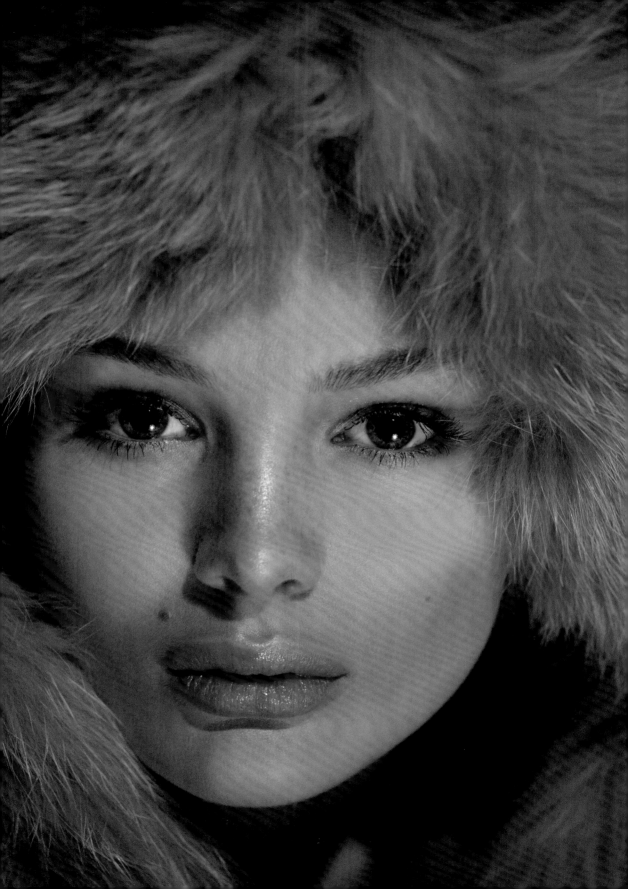

BONE BROTH

THE COLLAGEN DRINK

This may sound like some dodgy witch's brew – leftover bones boiled down in a big pot – yet it's so nutritious. It's just a grittier name for "stock," really, which I've been making for years to get the most out of a Sunday roast, but it also harks back to bygone times when people had to be thriftier, such as during the war, to make best use of the few ingredients on hand. They were on to something, though. Research in recent years has shown the importance of the gut for our immunity, so it stands to reason that bone broth – which is particularly helpful in healing the gut – is by extension good for our overall health. A great source of ingestible collagen, which supports hair, nail and skin health, and amino acids, which work to reduce inflammation, bone broth helps maintain the elasticity of the skin, keeping it looking smooth, youthful and clear. Its gut-healing properties aid the body's detoxification systems, too, ensuring clearer skin as a result. The perfect follow-up to a roast, bone broth/stock can be used as the basis for a wide range of dishes. It's ideal for making different soups, of course – such as my Hearty Chicken Soup (see p. 218) – adding greatly to their nutritional value.

SKIN-FEEDING NUTRIENTS

- Minerals:
  calcium
  magnesium
  phosphorus

- Protein:
  amino acids
    (arginine,
    glucosamine,
    glutamine,
    glycine, proline)
  collagen

CHICKEN BROTH (P. 228)

C ARROT

We humans have been eating carrots for thousands of years, and for good reason, too. A ready-made snack, carrots are both delicious and super nutritious; I love that they can be used raw in salads, cooked in roasts or grated into cakes – such a versatile vegetable, and increasingly available in a spectrum of different-colored heritage varieties, too. In fact, carrots are one of the richest sources of beta-carotene, which is an antioxidant that converts to vitamin A in the body, helping to repair aging skin tissue, as well as aid cellular turnover and protect skin from UV damage. There's even some truth in the old adage about carrots making you see in the dark: eating them may not endow you with superhero infrared vision, but vitamin A does protect the surface of your eyes, and therefore is important for their health. I love drinking carrot juice, too, especially to protect my skin from the sun, as it acts as a sort of internal sunscreen, although it's important to keep consumption to moderate levels or your skin can actually turn orange temporarily – not quite the "glowing" look we're going for! A source of vitamin C, carrots help the skin to look vibrant, plus it aids collagen production for overall skin maintenance and elasticity. Containing potassium, too, carrots can help to treat dry skin conditions, which are often linked to a deficiency of this mineral. Although carrots are a staple throughout the year, eating them in winter, when they're naturally in season, is thus particularly good for addressing skin issues of this kind.

SKIN-FEEDING NUTRIENTS

- Dietary fiber
- Minerals:
  copper
  iron
  potassium
- Phytochemicals:
  carotenoids
    (beta-carotene)

- Vitamins:
  A
  B6 (pyridoxine)
  B9 (folate)
  C
  E

HEARTY CHICKEN SOUP WITH CARROTS
AND SWEET POTATO (P. 218)

JERUSALEM ARTICHOKE

THE IRON BOOSTER

In case you're wondering, Jerusalem artichokes are completely different from the more familiar globe artichoke, with its edible fleshy leaves and heart. They're a root vegetable for a start – rather like a very small potato crossed with a ginger root. They don't look very inviting but they're super tasty: a mix between a potato, a parsnip and a turnip in flavor. They are a great alternative to potatoes – similar in texture but with a fresher taste that makes any dish feel "cleaner." Full of nutrients and dietary fiber, Jerusalem artichokes make an excellent addition to a varied skin-feeding diet. Particularly known for their high levels of iron, they can help reduce circles under the eyes, enliven a dull or pale complexion and improve energy levels. They're also a form of prebiotic, full of a nondigestible fiber known as inulin that stimulates the growth of "friendly" bacteria in the gut, as well as helps to fend off any of the bad bacteria, with additional benefits for the rest of the body. A source of potassium, they're great for maintaining a healthy blood pressure and for keeping the muscles working effectively. The copper in them helps in the production of collagen, while magnesium supports the detoxification pathways, including the skin, as well as being essential for healthy bones and teeth.

SKIN-FEEDING NUTRIENTS

- Dietary fiber:
  inulin
- Minerals:
  copper
  iron
  magnesium
  potassium
- Protein:
  amino acids
    (cysteine,
    methionine,
    taurine)

- Vitamins:
  B1 (thiamine)
  B2 (riboflavin)
  B3 (niacin)
  B5 (pantothenic acid)
  B6 (pyridoxine)
  B9 (folate)
  C

ROASTED JERUSALEM ARTICHOKES
AND MIXED ROOTS (P. 229)

K EFIR

Kefir is a fermented milk ingredient with a high concentration of helpful bacteria and yeasts that works to re-establish a healthy balance of flora and also to heal the damage caused by the overgrowth of "bad" bacteria. I can't rave enough about how important probiotics (and prebiotics – nondigestible fiber that helps support the good bacteria in the gut) are for the health of skin. Seriously – it all starts with the gut. Treating the gut for an imbalance in the flora will have a dramatic impact on the overall look and quality of the skin – not just in restoring a glow, but in treating more serious skin conditions like acne, eczema, rosacea and psoriasis, too. Suitable for those who are lactose-intolerant, kefir is also an excellent source of drinkable calcium, with one glass providing 20 percent of the daily recommended intake. Protein-rich, kefir is full of amino acids – essential for repairing skin cells and stimulating new growth. More potent than "live" yogurt for promoting "good" bacteria, kefir is made with a culture of so-called "kefir grains" – little clumps of bacteria and yeast that can be grown into a "live" drink with a thousand different health benefits. It may sound unappetizing, but actually it's a lively brew with a subtle flavor. Many people think they're doing the right thing when they opt for commercial fermented yogurt drinks, but unlike kefir these contain a huge amount of sugar (or sugar substitutes), and are often processed using heat, thus defeating the purpose of the gut-treating properties.

SKIN-FEEDING NUTRIENTS

- Minerals: calcium
- Probiotics
- Protein: amino acids (tryptophan)

COCONUT KEFIR (P. 236)

THE NATURAL DIURETIC

L EEK

One of the things I remember from reading *French Women Don't Get Fat* a few years back is that you should eat leek soup if you want to stay slim. The soup itself is filling, while leek is a diuretic, helping to get rid of any excess fluid in the body. So of course, from then on I made sure to include leeks in my diet. Containing silica and sulfur, among other skin-benefiting minerals, leeks help the body to keep collagen production fired up and the connective tissue supported for better elasticity. Along with garlic and onions, leeks help trap and flush away toxins, speeding up detoxification of the body and helping to keep the skin clear. The only way to promote radiance in the skin is to keep the body and the skin toxin-free and working well, making leeks an excellent skin-clearing food. Leeks are also a source of beta-carotene and vitamin C (especially in the greener parts of the plant), both powerful antioxidants that help protect skin against damage by free radicals and aging UV radiation, helping to keep the skin looking youthful.

SKIN-FEEDING NUTRIENTS

- Dietary fiber
- Minerals:
  calcium
  copper
  iron
  manganese
  phosphorus
  selenium
  silica
  sulfur
  zinc
- Phytochemicals:
  carotenoids (beta-
    carotene, lutein,
    zeaxanthin)

- Vitamins:
  A
  B1 (thiamine)
  B2 (riboflavin)
  B3 (niacin)
  B5 (pantothenic
  acid)
  B6 (pyridoxine)
  B9 (folate)
  C
  E
  K

HERBY LEEK AND PANCETTA PIZZAS (P. 216)

M ISO

A fermented food made from soybeans, miso has been consumed for thousands of years in both China and Japan, where it is known for its numerous benefits to health and beauty. You only have to take a walk through the streets of Japan to realize there must be some skincare secret – the women have the clearest, most luminous skin. I honestly believe it has to do with the Japanese diet, which is rich in fermented foods like miso and in iodine-rich seafood, while being low in dairy, gluten and refined sugar. While you've probably tried delicious Japanese foods like sushi, you may not realize how potent some of them are for the skin. Packed with antioxidants such as isoflavones, miso helps to address the signs of aging, while the fermented paste contains large amounts of beneficial bacteria that help the balance of flora in the gut, helping to keep the skin clear as a consequence. Working to strengthen the immune system, the alkalizing effect of miso helps keep the body strong and able to fight infection. The linoleic acid contained in miso is particularly good for the complexion – an essential fatty acid that helps keep the skin looking well nourished, clear and supple.

SKIN-FEEDING NUTRIENTS

- Dietary fiber
- Fatty acids:
  omega-6
    (linoleic acid)
- Minerals:
  calcium
- Phytochemicals:
  isoflavones
- Probiotics
- Protein:
  amino acids
    (tryptophan)

- Vitamins:
  B2 (riboflavin)
  B12 (cobalamin)
  choline
  E
  K

Mushroom

I've had spells in the past of not liking mushrooms, not because of the taste but on the assumption that, being a fungus, they weren't so good for you. Now I know better and can appreciate their nutritional value, especially for the skin. They are one of the only vegetables that can make vitamin D from sunlight, for instance. Essential for healthy bones and teeth, this nutrient also helps to regulate the turnover of skin cells, ensuring a radiant glow. The zinc in mushrooms stops you from producing too much sebum – or oil, in layman's terms – which in turn is great for the treatment of acne, the result of the body over-producing sebum. It used to be standard advice to peel off the skin of a mushroom, but this is where many of the nutrients are concentrated, so it's best left on for maximum nutritional benefit. I've never tried picking wild mushrooms because I'm always scared they might be poisonous. My Swedish friends pick them in droves, however, which might be why they're all so tall and have great skin.

SKIN-FEEDING NUTRIENTS

- Dietary fiber
- Minerals:
  copper
  magnesium
  manganese
  phosphorus
  potassium
  selenium
  zinc

- Vitamins:
  B2 (riboflavin)
  B3 (niacin)
  B12 (cobalamin)
  D

MUSHROOM FLATBREADS (P. 214)

Natural
Red Wine

THE YOUTH POTION

This might sound like wishful thinking, but including natural red wine in a skin-feeding diet is totally legit! The antioxidants it contains are quite potent when it comes to helping prevent premature aging of the skin. Of course that's not a license to drink a bottle a night – strict terms and conditions apply. It needs to be an occasional glass and a "natural" variety – made using organically grown grapes in a more traditional way and with no chemical additives or preservatives. Natural wines are increasingly sought after for this reason; they also have no added sugar, so there's no sugar hangover the next day. It's a simple and ancient approach to wine-making, particularly favored by the Italians, whose Mediterranean diet is famed for its health benefits. In particular, it's the powerful anti-aging antioxidant resveratrol in red wine that's said to slow the growth of acne-causing bacteria and fights disease-causing free radicals, making it especially useful for those who are acne-prone or suffering from an inflamed skin condition. Of course, I don't need any encouragement to have a glass of wine with dinner. (Though beware – natural wine does go down very easily, so that you can end up drinking more than you'd planned!) It's such a nice thing to share a glass with friends after a long day to accompany a beautifully cooked meal – one of the dishes in this book, naturally!

SKIN-FEEDING NUTRIENTS

- Phytochemicals:
polyphenols
  (resveratrol)

ONION

THE INFECTION FIGHTER

Someone once told me that if you pop a wooden spoon in your mouth when you're slicing an onion, it stops you from crying. I've never tried it. Donning sunglasses, another suggestion, would be more appealing – and a better look, it has to be said, though with reduced vision you might be weeping over a cut finger instead . . . We don't tend to think of the cooking staples like onions as being particularly nutritious. People use them as the basis for most savory dishes, chiefly for their flavor, forgetting that they are full of nutrients in their own right and therefore excellent as part of a healthy diet, with benefits to the skin, too. Helping to boost the circulation and fight disease, thanks to their natural antiviral properties, onions are particularly useful as a key ingredient in the winter months, when your immune system can face increased challenges. Their anti-inflammatory properties mean they help the body to stay strong and defend itself against infection, while the nondigestible fiber they contain encourages the good bacteria in the gut to flourish and keep it healthy, ensuring the proper absorption of nutrients and elimination of waste. This in turn will be reflected in your skin, enabling it to stay clear and with a healthy glow. Meanwhile, the vitamins C and E in onions support the skin's collagen and protect it from UV damage – making onions an excellent wrinkle-fighting food you can easily incorporate in your diet. Luckily the nutrients in onions are not as impaired by heat as they are in other foods, which is helpful given that we tend to eat them cooked in dishes.

SKIN-FEEDING NUTRIENTS

- Dietary fiber
- Minerals:
  iron
  potassium
  sulfur
- Phytochemicals:
  allicin

- Vitamins:
  B6 (pyridoxine)
  B9 (folate)
  C
  E

FRENCH ONION SOUP (P. 210)

ORANGE

I love the smell and zingy taste of oranges – is there anything more refreshing? They are the embodiment of vitamin C for most people, and for good reason, too, as this nutrient plays a crucial role in strengthening the immune system. Oranges are packed with vitamin C, so it makes sense to up your intake of the fruit when the weather gets chillier and to help fend off colds and bugs. Vitamin C helps the body to absorb plant-based iron and it's also needed for the production of collagen, a vital component in the structure and elasticity of the skin. Oranges have a broad spectrum of other nutritional benefits: their fiber content means it's best to eat them just as they are – the detoxifying pectin (a form of soluble fiber) they contain helps to keep the digestive system moving, eliminating waste for a clearer colon and less congested skin. It's always better to include all of the flesh of the fruit to reap the benefits of the fiber and slow down absorption of the sugar in the juice. I always avoid drinking orange juice for this reason, as it can be too much sugar on the system in one hit, causing blood sugar to spike.

SKIN-FEEDING NUTRIENTS

- Dietary fiber: pectin
- Minerals: calcium potassium
- Phytochemicals: flavonoids polyphenols

- Vitamins: B1 (thiamine) B6 (pyridoxine) B9 (folate) C

THE PLANT-BASED POWER FOOD

P
UY LENTIL

Puy lentils are another one of those ingredients that people write off as "hippie" food, but nutritionally they pack a real punch and they're great for the skin, too. Originating in the Le Puy region of France, with its rich volcanic soil, Puy lentils are earthy and nutty-textured. Loaded with plant-based protein, they work to stabilize blood-sugar levels and release their energy slowly. This is crucial for the beauty of the skin, as it's very sensitive to the roller-coaster of energy highs and lows, and can become inflamed when the body is subjected to blood-sugar spikes. They're super rich in folate, too, essential for cellular repair and therefore an excellent anti-aging nutrient. Their high iron content also helps with energy levels and to give luster and life to skin, hair and nails. The radiance-boosting vitamin C works to protect the skin from UV light, targeting existing sun damage as well. Meanwhile, the soluble fiber in Puy lentils makes them hugely beneficial to the digestive tract – if the gut and colon are clear and functioning well, this helps the skin, as less pressure is put on it to eliminate waste products that have built up elsewhere in the body. The lentil stew I've included here provides nearly half your daily intake of zinc, which helps to regulate the production of sebum, whether your skin is oily or dry.

SKIN-FEEDING NUTRIENTS

- Dietary fiber
- Minerals:
  copper
  manganese
  phosphorus
  zinc
- Protein
- Vitamins:
  B1 (thiamine)
  B6 (pyridoxine)
  B9 (folate)
  C

CHICKEN AND PUY LENTIL STEW (P. 222)

RED CABBAGE

If there's one thing I've learned about nutrition for the skin it's that you can never have too much vitamin C–rich food; it's the number one nutrient for collagen-building and for brightening the complexion. And although you might not have expected it, red cabbage is packed to the rafters with vitamin C, which works to impart that incredible glow that very healthy people have. I always choose red cabbage over green for that reason, as it has almost twice the amount of vitamin C – and in my opinion a better flavor, too. Other essential nutrients in red cabbage are also potent in the treatment and repair of the skin. Working to hydrate from within like an internal moisturizer, they help the complexion look supple, smooth and nourished. Fiber-rich and low in calories, red cabbage is a great digestive aid – the roughage helps eliminate waste from the gut, while also helping you to feel full. The deep purple tint of red cabbage comes from the carotenoids it contains. These act as an anti-inflammatory in the body, making red cabbage an excellent beauty treatment for fighting inflammation-based skin problems like psoriasis and eczema.

SKIN-FEEDING NUTRIENTS

- Dietary fiber
- Minerals:
  calcium
  manganese
  phosphorus
  potassium
  sulfur
  zinc
- Phytochemicals:
  carotenoids
  (alpha- and beta-
  carotene, lutein,
  zeaxanthin)

- Vitamins:
  B5 (pantothenic
  acid)
  B6 (pyridoxine)
  B9 (folate)
  C
  K

RHUBARB

THE FIBER-RICH FAVORITE

My best friend was over for dinner one night and said "yes" to a dessert, but then didn't eat it. When I asked her why, she replied: "I hate rhubarb." This was years ago, but just recently she told me that she discovered she's lacking in magnesium, which is ironic because if she'd been eating rhubarb all that time, it might have helped! Rhubarb contains magnesium, which is especially good for your skin and for reducing the build-up of lactic acid in the muscles after a workout. It is also high in fiber and acts as a natural laxative, so it is great for digestion and weight loss, too. In addition, rhubarb has antibacterial and antifungal properties, helping to reduce inflammation and treat infection. Its sweetness is countered by a more complex tart taste, making it the perfect ingredient for a rustic dessert. It's actually a vegetable, not a fruit.

SKIN-FEEDING NUTRIENTS

- Dietary fiber
- Minerals:
  calcium
  copper
  magnesium
  manganese
  potassium
  selenium

- Vitamins:
  B1 (thiamine)
  B2 (riboflavin)
  B3 (niacin)
  B5 (pantothenic acid)
  B9 (folate)
  C
  K

GLUTEN-FREE RHUBARB CRUMBLE (P. 232)

ROSEMARY

THE SKIN ENERGIZER

Rosemary has such an amazing smell and taste. The oils in the rosemary plant are so fragrant you hardly need to touch it to release its gorgeous aroma. One of the most common herbs, rosemary is one of those grow-everywhere plants that people take for granted, but it's a powerful herb that works to treat the body and skin in many ways. It's naturally astringent and has anti-inflammatory properties, which is why you'll often find it as an active ingredient in many skincare products. Helping to reduce redness and puffiness, rosemary also works to address breakouts that come from excess sebum production, making it an excellent addition to the diet for anyone with skin problems like congested pores or acne. Rosemary is known for its ability to stimulate circulation, giving a more lustrous complexion and helping internal systems to function more effectively. The powerful fragrance that comes from the rosemary leaves is more than just an added bonus; the scent is thought to improve mood (it may help to decrease levels of the stress hormone cortisol), boost energy and enhance brain function, too – which is never a bad thing. Used topically – I like to use a few drops in a bath – rosemary essential oil helps to treat indigestion, excess gas and menstrual disorders, as well as promoting mental clarity and relieving mental fatigue. Used in cooking, its wide range of nutrients and vitamins can improve elasticity of the skin and stimulate cell turnover – adding to that sought-after glow. Rosemary keeps well after being cut, for at least 5 days in the fridge; I like to keep my cut herbs in a glass of water to keep them alive even longer.

SKIN-FEEDING NUTRIENTS

- Dietary fiber
- Fatty acids:
  omega-3
- Minerals:
  calcium
  iron
  magnesium
  manganese
  zinc
- Vitamins:
  A
  C

ROSEMARY TEA (P. 236)

THE SEED OF IMMORTALITY

SESAME SEED

Sesame seeds have been prized by the Chinese for centuries (and by early Hindu tradition, too), known to them as the "seed of immortality," in the belief that they can promote longevity and beauty – at any age. Their high protein and rich oil content makes them ideal for those looking for good plant-based sources of protein and other essential nutrients that are also full of flavor. While white sesame seeds are commonly used in cooking in Middle Eastern dishes (as well as ground up in a paste to make tahini) and increasingly in the West, the black seeds are less well known, though both types are equally nutritious and recommended for any skin-feeding diet. For such a tiny foodstuff, sesame seeds contain an incredible array of potent actives that work to keep your skin looking younger for longer. Known to treat the signs of aging – thinning or gray hair and wrinkles – they also strengthen bones and promote good vision. If you buy a bag of these for a particular recipe, they shouldn't sit in the pantry unused, as they can be sprinkled on to any meal, salad or smoothie to enhance the flavor and some gorgeous nutty texture.

SKIN-FEEDING NUTRIENTS

- Dietary fiber
- Fatty acids:
  omega-3
  omega-6
    (linoleic acid)
- Minerals:
  calcium
  magnesium
  phosphorus
  potassium
  zinc
- Protein
- Vitamins
  B1 (thiamine)
  B2 (riboflavin)
  B3 (niacin)
  B6 (pyridoxine)
  B9 (folate)

BLACK SESAME STIR-FRY (P. 220)

TOFU

THE PLANT-BASED PROTEIN

Soy products like tofu come with a fair bit of controversy attached – some people love them, some people hate them. In the "no" camp are those who say the soybean is grown using destructive methods and with excessive use of pesticides – which is why choosing organic tofu is so important, quite apart from being nutritionally better for you. There's also the argument that the phytoestrogens in tofu can lead to hormonal imbalance in both men and women, although the verdict is still out on this. In the "yes" camp are those (including every vegetarian I know) who will defend tofu to the hilt. And there are plenty of good reasons for eating it – providing it is organic, of course – the main one being the huge skin-feeding benefits that come with both tofu and tempeh, its fermented (and arguably healthier) cousin. Full of plant-based protein that improves the elasticity of the skin, helping to keep it taut and supple, tofu is also rich in minerals, making tofu an excellent meat alternative for vegetarians or those looking to cut down on meat.

SKIN-FEEDING NUTRIENTS

- Fatty acids:
  omega-3
- Minerals:
  calcium
  copper
  iron
  manganese
  phosphorus
  selenium

- Phytochemicals:
  phytoestrogens

THE LOW-CAL ROOT

Turnip

Like most people, I absolutely love root vegetables in winter. There's something so comforting about a roasted potato or turnip – crispy on the outside and fluffy on the inside – especially when the weather turns cold. But unlike potatoes, whose starch and carbohydrate content converts to sugar quite quickly in the body, turnips have all of the comforting qualities without the inevitable blood-sugar spikes and slumps. Surprisingly low in calories but high in fiber, turnips help to regulate the metabolism and support the gut for more efficient detoxification, all of which makes them a great choice when looking to control weight through diet. Turnips are also rich in glucosinolates, a natural component of many bitter plants that help the stomach get rid of "bad bacteria" and improves the health of the gut, and the skin by extension. Brilliant for directly feeding the complexion, turnips are known for their anti-aging properties, mostly due to high levels of antioxidant vitamins and phytochemicals and because they are packed full of minerals. They are also handy when making a snowman and you need a nose, for a more stylish alternative to a carrot!

SKIN-FEEDING NUTRIENTS

- Dietary fiber
- Minerals:
  calcium
  manganese
  phosphorus
  potassium
- Phytochemicals:
  carotenoids (lutein)
  glucosinolates

- Vitamins:
  B1 (thiamine)
  B5 (pantothenic acid)
  B6 (pyridoxine)
  B9 (folate)
  C

CLASSIC ROAST CHICKEN WITH TURNIPS (P. 230)

THE BRAIN AND SKIN FOOD

WHITE FISH

White fish constitute a big part of my diet. Although lower in omega-3 fatty acids than their oily counterparts – such as salmon and sardines (see pp. 47 and 154) – they have the advantage of being lower in fat as well as high in protein. I often eat white fish for dinner for this reason, knowing the lean protein won't weigh me down during the night. I always try to buy line-caught rather than farmed fish to avoid the growth hormones and antibiotics they are fed. The more organic or natural the rearing process, the better. Most people associate fish with good health – and it stands to reason. You only have to look at those cultures that consume a lot of fresh fish to see greater evidence of heart health and longevity; and arguably people who eat lots of fish have improved brain function, too. While the nutritional profile of specific species will be slightly different, there are nutritional benefits they all have in common. For a start, fish is a good source of essential fatty acids like omega-3, which reduce inflammation, improving pretty much every system in the body – and especially the skin. I have to say, when I've been exercising a lot, and a joint might be sore, if I've taken an omega-3, 6 and 9 tablet, it will improve the injury within a day or so. Inflammation can cause the skin cells to clog the pores, leading to conditions like acne, which is why eating fish is so helpful for keeping the skin clear and congestion-free. Rich in selenium – an antioxidant mineral that both protects skin from sun damage and helps to repair existing damage – fish is a powerful protector owing to this nutrient, which works to maintain the firmness and elasticity of the skin.

SKIN-FEEDING NUTRIENTS

- Fatty acids:
  omega-3
  omega-6
- Minerals:
  phosphorus
  potassium
  selenium
- Protein:
  all nine essential
    amino acids
- Vitamins:
  B1 (thiamine)
  B2 (riboflavin)
  B3 (niacin)
  B6 (pyridoxine)
  B12 (cobalamin)

Miso
soup

SERVES 4

————

30 CALORIES
PER SERVING

————

- 5 strips of wakame (seaweed)
- 5 cups still mineral water
- 1 shallot, thinly sliced
- 2 tbsp miso paste
- 2 oz tofu or tempeh,
  cut into small cubes
- Sea salt or tamari

TO GARNISH (OPTIONAL)
- Scallions, chopped
- Fresh chives, snipped
- Watercress
- Dried crushed red pepper
  flakes
- Grated fresh ginger

This is great for a fasting day or to have as a drink if you're busy, just to tide you over. Customize it depending on what you have in the fridge. As long as you have miso paste – preferably a good-quality, organic (non-GMO) brand – you have the basis for so many different versions of the soup.

1. Soak the wakame in the mineral water for 10 minutes and cut into 1-inch strips.
2. Place the wakame and its soaking water in a large pan with the shallot and bring to a boil. Reduce the heat and simmer for 10–20 minutes or until tender.
3. Transfer 1½ cups of broth from the saucepan into a bowl. Allow the broth in the bowl to cool a little, then stir in the miso. (The broth should not be boiling, as it could kill the live bacteria and enzymes in the miso.)
4. Pour the miso mixture into the soup in the pan, then add the tofu or tempeh and season to taste with sea salt or tamari. Serve with your choice of garnish.

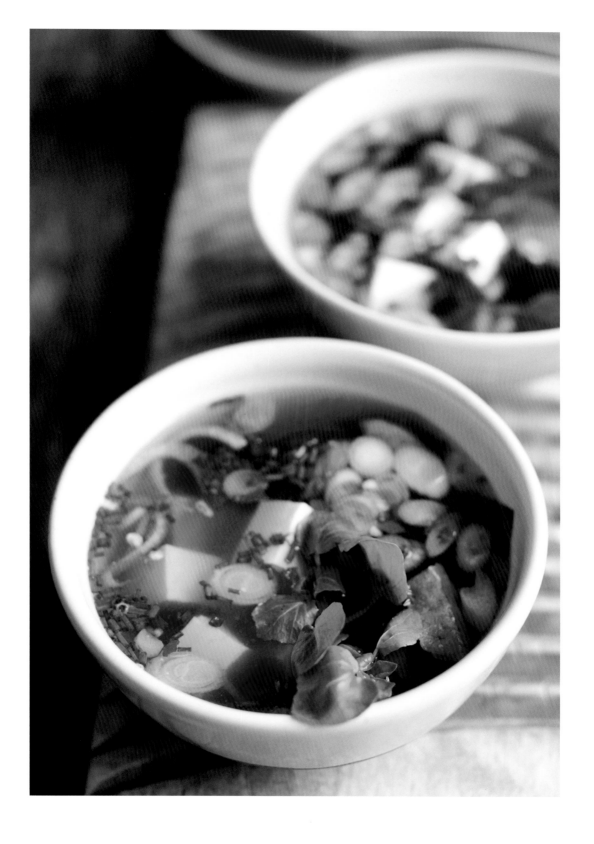

French onion soup

SERVES 4

————

245 CALORIES
PER SERVING

————

- 1 tbsp olive oil
- 2 tbsp butter
- 1½ lbs onions (about
  5 medium onions),
  thinly sliced in rings
- 3 garlic cloves,
  finely chopped
- 5 cups vegetable stock
- 2 tbsp apple cider vinegar
- Sea salt and black pepper

I really got into this soup when I was living in Paris – the French swear by it for treating hangovers! I've omitted the croutons and Gruyère included in the classic version for a lighter dish.

1. Place the oil and butter in a large pan set over high heat. Once melted, add the onions and garlic. Sauté for 5 minutes or until the onions are tinged with brown.
2. Reduce the heat to low and cook, stirring occasionally, for 30 minutes. By then, the base of the pan should be covered in a rich, nut-brown, caramelized film.
3. Pour in the stock and vinegar and stir in well, scrape the bottom of the pan to incorporate the caramelized onions. Bring to a simmer, then turn down the heat and leave for 1 hour. Season before pouring into bowls.

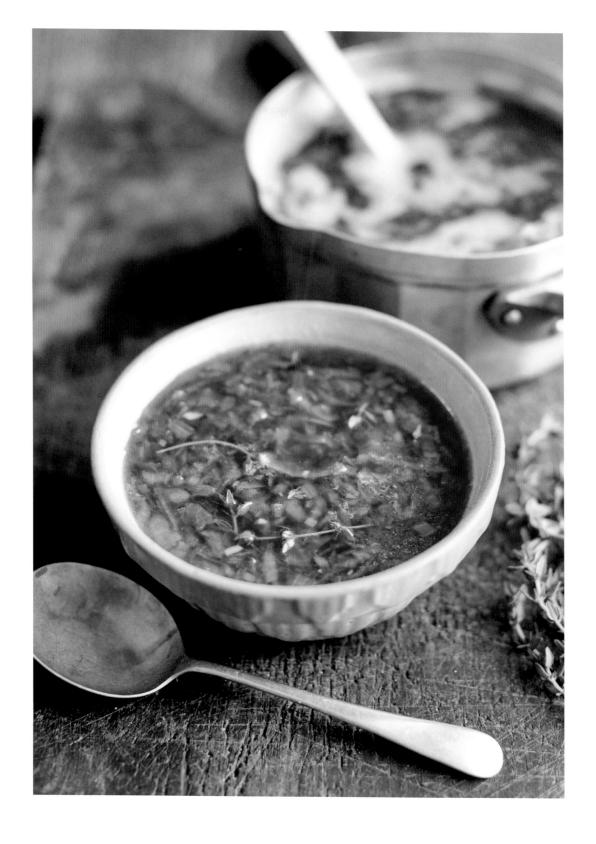

Red cabbage salad

SERVES 2

———

183 CALORIES
PER SERVING

———

- 1 carrot, finely sliced
- 1 green apple (unpeeled), cored and finely sliced
- 1–4 red cabbage, finely sliced
- 1 tbsp sliced almonds
- 1 piece of broccolini, finely sliced

FOR THE DRESSING

- 1 tbsp extra-virgin olive oil
- 1 tbsp apple cider vinegar
- 1 tsp chopped fresh dill
- 1–2 tsp celery seeds
- 1–4 tsp ground turmeric
- 1–4 tsp paprika
- 1–2 tsp sea salt
- 1–2 tsp ground black pepper

Have you heard of the paleo diet? It's all about eating as the early humans might have done – so lots of meat, fish, vegetables and fruit and no cereals, dairy or processed foods. This is essentially a paleo recipe, being mostly vegetables and a little fruit. The red cabbage is the key ingredient for your skin, though the apple and carrot are beneficial, too, and broccolini is a good source of complexion-clearing vitamin B2. The salad is a favorite of mine – a dairy-free take on coleslaw, traditionally made with white cabbage. The red cabbage both looks better, in my view, and is much nicer to eat raw.

1. Place the carrot, apple, cabbage, almonds and broccolini in a bowl.
2. Place the ingredients for the dressing in a small jar or bowl and stir well before pouring over the chopped salad ingredients and mixing together thoroughly.

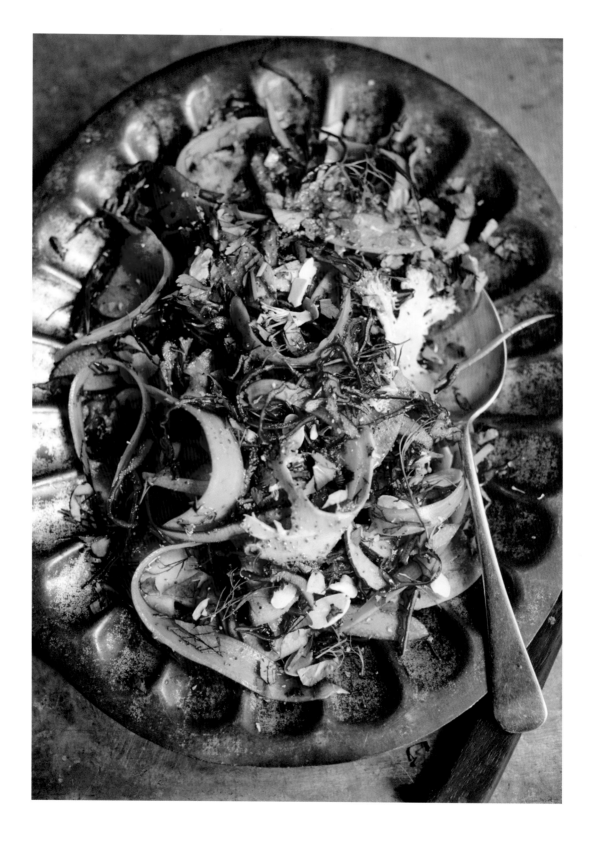

Mushroom flatbreads

SERVES 2

———

140 CALORIES
PER SERVING

———

- 1 tsp raw coconut oil
- 2 shallots, finely chopped
- 2 garlic cloves, crushed
- 2 handfuls of mushrooms, roughly chopped
- 2 tbsp crème fraîche or coconut milk
- ½ oz Parmesan cheese, finely grated, plus extra to serve
- 2 handfuls of baby spinach
- Flat-leaf parsley, finely chopped
- Sea salt and black pepper
- 2 buckwheat flatbreads (see p. 160), to serve

Mushrooms, with their earthy taste and fleshy texture, make a really good alternative to meat, especially when they're cooked the right way – you don't feel as though you're missing out. On my vegetarian days, I love to bake mushrooms whole – eating a big one can be just like eating a piece of meat. For this recipe, you can use any mushrooms you like – either a mixture or just one kind. Whatever suits.

1. Melt the coconut oil in a large sauté pan; add the shallots and garlic and cook over medium heat for 2 minutes.
2. Add the mushrooms to the pan, then lower the heat and cook for about 5 minutes or until most of the water released from the mushrooms has evaporated.
3. Add the crème fraîche or coconut milk to the pan with the Parmesan and stir in before seasoning well with salt and pepper.
4. Throw in the baby spinach and cook for 2–3 minutes or until just softened – it doesn't need to wilt down completely – then add the chopped parsley to the pan.
5. Serve on top of the buckwheat flatbreads, garnished with extra Parmesan.

MUSHROOM (P. 196)

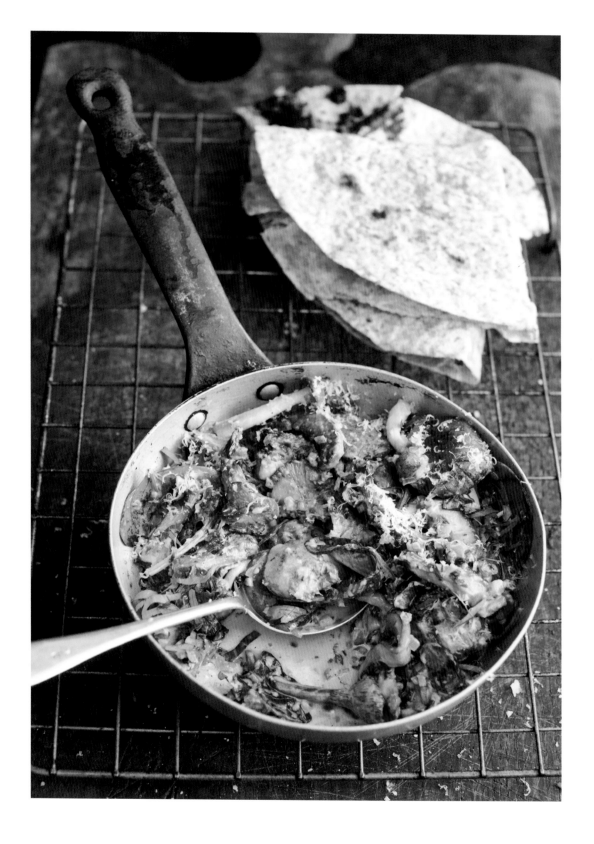

Herby leek and pancetta pizzas

MAKES 4 SMALL PIZZAS

———

1,026 CALORIES
PER PIZZA

———

FOR THE TOMATO SAUCE
- 1 tbsp olive oil
- 1 medium onion, finely chopped
- 1 garlic clove, finely chopped
- 2 (14½-oz) cans of chopped cherry tomatoes
- 1 tsp dried oregano
- 1 tsp dried basil
- 1 tsp honey
- Fine sea salt and black pepper

FOR THE PIZZA DOUGH
- 2½ cups tepid water
- 3 (¼-oz) sachets of dried yeast, or 1 oz fresh yeast
- 2 tbsp honey
- 8 cups strong bread flour, plus extra for dusting
- 1 level tbsp salt

I cook a lot with leeks in the winter, including that much-vaunted leek soup! Here I've used them as a topping for pizza – the perfect thing for an indulgent movie night. The leeks flush out any toxins. The canned tomatoes provide a good source of the antioxidants lycopene and beta-carotene, each with a protective effect on the skin and better absorbed in the presence of oil. This is the only recipe that has wheat in it – a treat.

1. First make the sauce. Heat the oil in a large high-sided skillet; add the onion and garlic and fry over medium heat for 5 minutes or until soft. Add the tomatoes and simmer over a low heat for 40 minutes or until thickened.
2. Add the dried herbs and honey, then season to taste with salt and pepper before setting aside.
3. While the sauce is cooking, make the dough. Pour half the water into a bowl and add the yeast and honey, leaving it for 3 minutes for the honey to dissolve.
4. Place the flour and the salt in a large bowl and create a well in the middle. Pour the yeast mixture into the well.
5. Start to bring the flour in from outside the well. Continue doing this until the center of the mixture is porridge-like in consistency, then add the remaining water. Mix again, continuing to bring in flour from the edge of the bowl until fully incorporated.
6. On a work surface lightly dusted in flour, start to knead the dough by pushing and folding it on itself. Roll it around, over and over, for 4–5 minutes or until the dough is smooth and elastic in consistency.
7. Place the dough in a large clean bowl, sprinkle over a little flour, then cover in plastic wrap and allow it to rise for half an hour. It should double in size.
8. Shortly before the dough has finished rising, preheat the oven to 475°F and lightly dust 2–4 baking sheets with flour.
9. Place the leek in a small pan of boiling water and blanch for 3 minutes. Drain well and set aside.

    LEEK (P. 194)

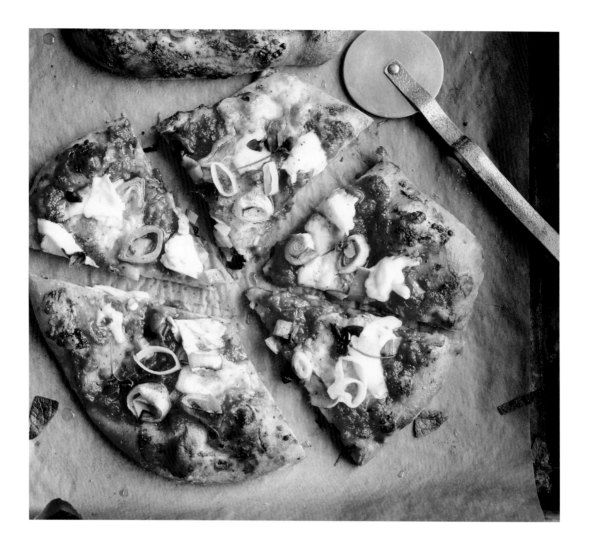

FOR THE PIZZA TOPPING
- 1 leek, sliced into short lengths
- Olive oil, for drizzling
- 3½ oz buffalo mozzarella, cut into pieces
- 2½ oz sliced unsmoked pancetta, torn into pieces
- Leaves from 1 sprig of rosemary

10. When the dough has finished proving, knock the air out for 30 seconds by squashing it on a flour-dusted work surface. Divide into four balls, then roll out on into disks about 1 inch thick and 8 inches in diameter.

11. Transfer the pizza bases to the prepared baking sheets. Spread each pizza base with tomato sauce (see tip below) and drizzle a little olive oil over the edges.

12. Top each pizza with the mozzarella, then divide the leek, pancetta and rosemary between the pizzas and bake in the oven – in two batches, if necessary – for 8–10 minutes.

TIP
- You'll most likely have a bit of the sauce left over; don't overload the dough or it will become soggy.

Hearty chicken soup with carrots and sweet potato

SERVES 2

————

400 CALORIES
PER SERVING

————

- 2 tsp raw coconut oil
- 1 medium onion, diced
- 2 garlic cloves, finely chopped
- 4 celery stalks, diced
- 2½ cups chicken stock (to make your own, see p. 228)
- 2 skinless and boneless chicken breasts, diced
- 4 pieces of broccolini, florets separated and stems cut into small pieces
- 1 sweet potato, peeled and diced
- ¾ cup peas
- 2 carrots, diced
- Sea salt and black pepper
- Small handful of flat-leaf parsley, finely chopped, to serve

During cold and flu season there's nothing better than a warming bowl of chicken soup – truly "food for the soul" – made with homemade chicken broth (preferably) and full of nutritious vegetables to help the body to heal itself. I love this recipe and I cook it when I want to feel warm and cozy. It is a real favorite with all my friends, too: I tend to make a big pot and freeze any that's left over (though there rarely is). The nutrients in the carrots – along with the medicinal qualities of the chicken broth (see p. 141) – may help to reduce cold symptoms in the upper respiratory tract, with other ingredients all working to help make you feel human again.

1. Melt the coconut oil in a large saucepan over low heat. Add the onion, garlic and celery, cover the pan with a lid and sweat the vegetables for 5–7 minutes or until translucent.
2. Season with salt and pepper and pour in the stock.
3. Add the chicken, chopped broccolini stalks and three-quarters of the sweet potato, then bring to a simmer and cook, uncovered, for 15 minutes.
4. Add 1¼ cups of water and throw in the rest of the sweet potato, the broccolini florets and all the remaining vegetables. Bring back up to a simmer and cook for 20–30 minutes.
5. Taste for seasoning and divide the soup between bowls, scattering with chopped parsley to serve.

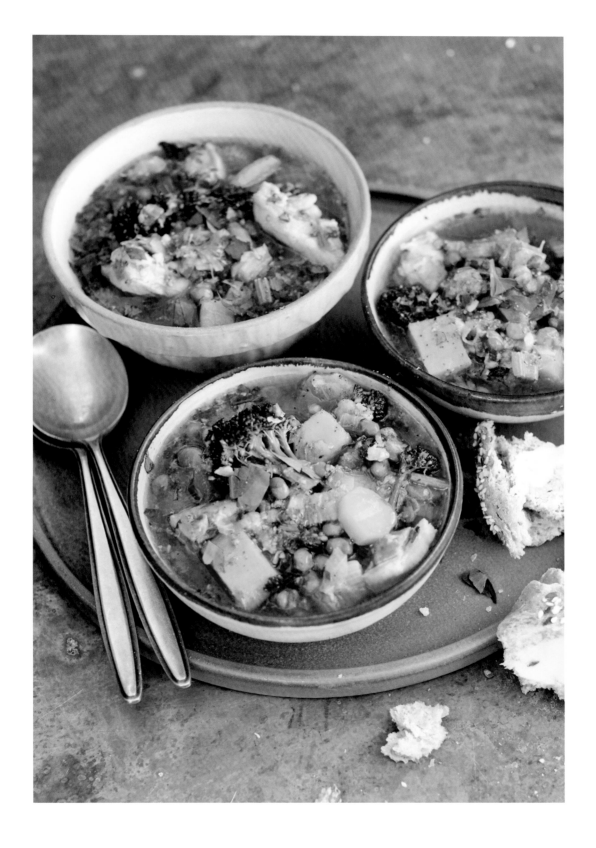

Black sesame stir-fry

SERVES 2

———

490 CALORIES
PER SERVING

———

FOR THE MARINADE
- 1 fresh red chile, seeded and finely chopped
- 1 garlic clove, finely chopped
- Small handful of fresh cilantro, chopped, plus extra to garnish
- 1 tbsp honey
- 1-inch knob of fresh ginger, peeled and finely grated
- Juice of ½ lime
- 1 tbsp tamari

- 2 skinless and boneless chicken breasts, diced
- 1 tbsp raw coconut oil
- 2 carrots, sliced
- 4 scallions, sliced
- 4 pieces of broccolini, cut into pieces
- Handful of snow peas, sliced
- Handful of bean sprouts
- Juice of ½ lime
- 1 tbsp tamari

TO GARNISH
- Handful of raw peanuts, crushed
- 1 tbsp black sesame seeds

This healthy stir-fry has just the right amount of spiciness and crunch – with all the skin-feeding nutrients your complexion needs during the winter months, including high amounts of the antioxidant beta-carotene that can be found in the carrots and green veggies. This essential nutrient can accumulate in the fatty subcutaneous layer below the skin surface and protect against free-radical damage.

1. Place all the marinade ingredients in a bowl. Add the chicken to the marinade and set aside in the refrigerator for 20 minutes.
2. Melt the coconut oil in a large skillet or wok and add the marinated chicken. Stir-fry over medium heat for 10 minutes.
3. Add the carrots, scallions, broccolini, snow peas and bean sprouts to the pan, along with the lime juice and 1 tablespoon of water, and cover with a lid. Cook for 5 minutes, giving the pan a shake from time to time, and add the tamari.
4. Remove the pan from the heat and serve the stir-fry garnished with the peanuts, black sesame seeds and fresh cilantro

TIP
- For a vegetarian option, replace the chicken with tofu.

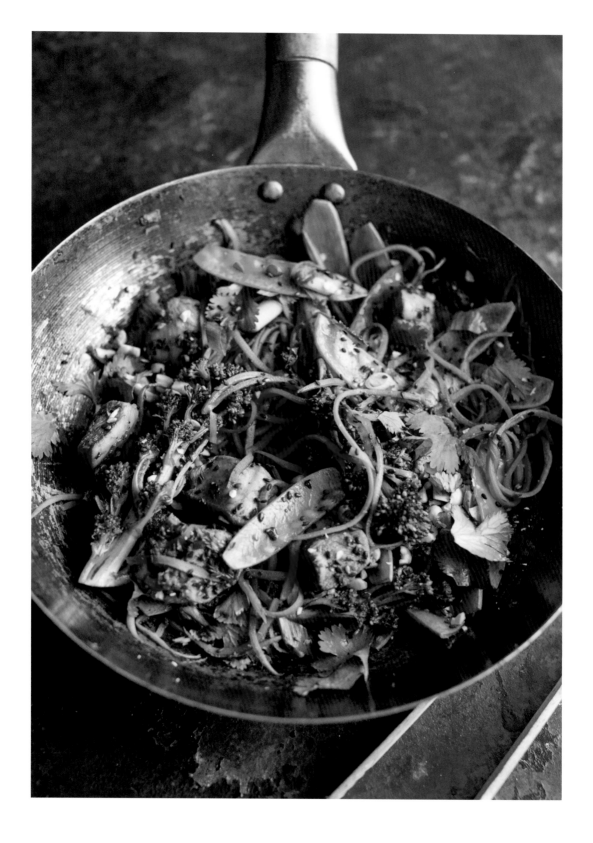

Chicken and
Puy lentil stew

SERVES 4

————

453 CALORIES
PER SERVING

————

- 1 tbsp olive oil
- 4 chicken thighs and
  4 chicken drumsticks
  (skin left on)
- 1 red onion, thinly sliced
- 2 garlic cloves, crushed
- 8 oz dried Puy lentils,
  rinsed
- 3¼ cups hot chicken stock
  (to make your own, see
  p. 228)
- 1 tbsp coconut milk
- Juice and grated zest
  of ½ lemon
- 1 tbsp Dijon mustard
- Small bunch of fresh
  parsley, chopped
- Sea salt and black pepper

I like the Puy variety of lentils best, as they hold their shape when cooked – ideal for dishes like this stew or a lentil-based salad. Other varieties tend to go a bit mushy, though that's perfect for making something like a dhal. This recipe is such a warming and hearty dish for the winter months: its abundance of iron and protein means everyone is left feeling happy and full, while the nutrients are left to work their magic on the skin – a win-win situation. Serve with a green salad, if desired.

1. Pour the olive oil into a large saucepan or flameproof casserole dish over high heat. Season the chicken pieces with salt and pepper, then brown in the hot oil for about 3 minutes each side or until golden all over. Remove from the pan and set aside, pouring away all but 1 tablespoon of oil left in the pan.
2. Add the onion to the pan and cook over medium heat for 5 minutes or until softened, then add the garlic and cook for a further minute.
3. Add the lentils and stock and stir well. Place the cooked chicken pieces on top, cover with a lid and leave to simmer over medium heat for 30 minutes. Remove the lid and increase the heat, then cook for another 20 minutes or until the lentils are tender, most of the stock has been absorbed and the chicken is cooked through.
4. Stir in the coconut milk, lemon juice and zest, mustard and parsley. Season to taste with salt and pepper and divide between plates, allowing one thigh and one drumstick per person.

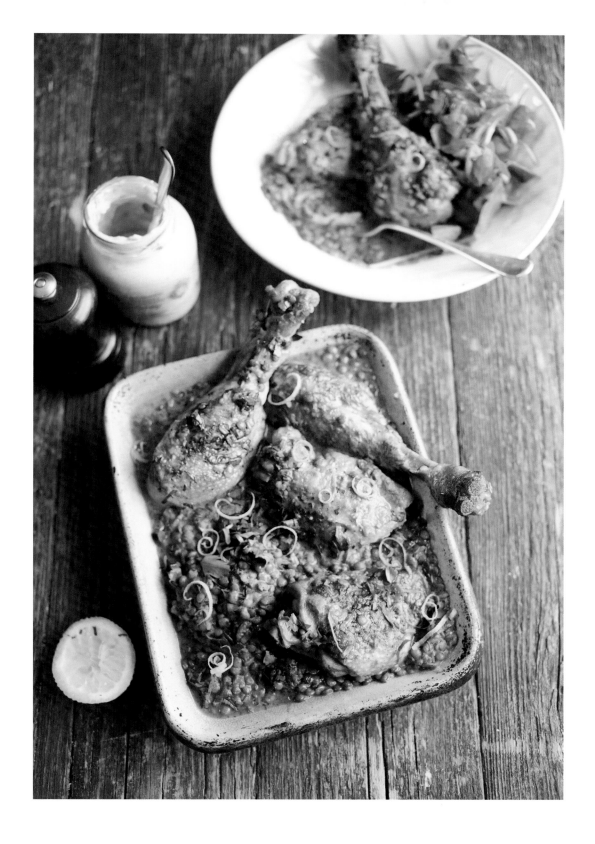

Naked
fish pie

SERVES 4

___

340 CALORIES
PER SERVING

___

- 2 large sweet potatoes,
  peeled and cut
  into small chunks
- 2 tbsp butter
- ¼ cup gluten-free flour
- 1¼ cups 1% milk (see tip
  below), warmed
- Juice of ½ lemon
- 1¼ cups vegetable stock
- 1 tsp whole-grain mustard
- 2 tbsp grated Parmesan cheese
- 1 lb white fish fillets
  (such as cod, hake,
  haddock and pollock),
  cut into chunks
- 1 small fennel bulb,
  halved and thinly sliced
- Sea salt and black pepper

I love eating fish – as well as being highly nutritious, it's speedy to cook. The only downside is the smell when you cook it, which is why I always end up baking it in foil or putting it in a pie. Warming and tasty – and including different types of white fish for a wider range of nutrients – this pie is perfect for the winter. The sweet potatoes I've used for the topping are a rich source of beta-carotene. Converted to vitamin A in the body, it helps to treat acne as it regulates the secretion of sebum and improves skin tone.

1. Preheat the oven to 425°F.
2. Place the potatoes in a large pan filled with water and boil for 10 minutes or until tender. Drain before mashing with a potato masher, adding salt and pepper to taste.
3. Meanwhile, make a white sauce by first melting the butter in a medium saucepan over medium heat. Add the flour and stir for about 2 minutes or until a paste forms. Next, slowly add the milk, stirring all the while, until you have a smooth sauce. Continue to stir the sauce for a further 5–10 minutes until it thickens.
4. Add the lemon juice to the sauce, followed by the stock and mustard. Season to taste with salt and pepper and stir in 1 teaspoon of Parmesan. Bring to a simmer and cook for 1 minute before removing from the heat.
5. Place the fish in a medium ovenproof dish with the sliced fennel. Pour over the white sauce and top with the sweet potato mash. Sprinkle the remaining Parmesan over the top.
6. Place the dish on a baking sheet. Transfer to the oven for 40 minutes or until cooked through and golden. Serve immediately.

TIP
- You can replace the 1% milk with coconut milk to lend a more Southeast Asian flavor to the fish.
- To round out the meal, serve with a green vegetable such as spinach, kale or broccoli.

WHITE FISH (P. 207)

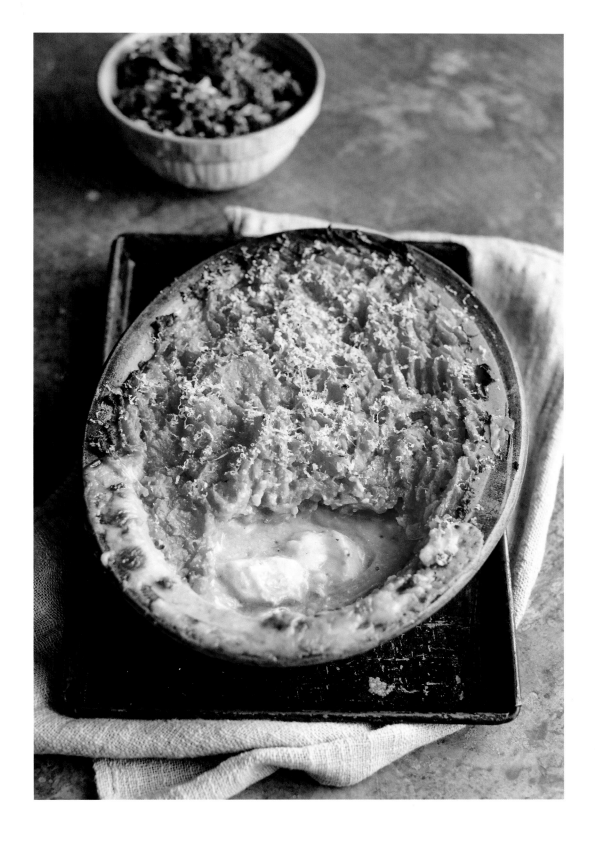

Spicy noodle soup with tofu

SERVES 2

————

610 CALORIES
PER SERVING

————

FOR THE SPICE PASTE
- 1-inch knob of fresh ginger, peeled and grated
- 2 lemongrass stalks (outer leaves removed), chopped
- 2 fresh red chiles, seeded and chopped, plus extra to garnish
- 3 shallots, chopped
- 1 garlic clove, finely chopped
- 1 tsp ground turmeric
- Pinch of sea salt
- 1 tbsp coconut oil

- 14 oz udon noodles
- 13½ oz can of coconut milk
- 1 cup vegetable stock
- 1 tsp coconut oil
- 20 oyster mushrooms, finely sliced
- 8 sugar snap peas, halved
- 6 oz fresh tofu, cut into 1-inch squares and dried on paper towels

TO GARNISH
- Fresh cilantro leaves
- Crushed raw peanuts
- Bean sprouts
- Lime wedges

I love adding cubes of tofu to a noodle soup like this one: the gluten-free noodles and protein are sustaining, making me feel full, while the soup itself is full of gorgeous flavor from the chile, turmeric and lemongrass. It's a recipe that offers a wonderfully warming, nutritious meal in the colder winter months – a great alternative for vegetarians, plus a boost to the beauty of the skin as well.

1. Place all the ingredients for the spice paste in a food processor and blend to a pulp. Set aside.
2. Cook the udon noodles in a large saucepan of boiling water according to the package instructions and set aside to drain.
3. Place a medium skillet over medium heat, add the spice paste and fry for 2–3 minutes. Pour in the coconut milk and vegetable stock and bring to a boil. Reduce the heat and simmer for 5 minutes.
4. Heat the coconut oil in a separate large skillet over medium heat. Add the oyster mushrooms and fry for 3 minutes or until softened.
5. Add the mushrooms to the sauce in the first skillet. Add the sugar snap peas, tofu and drained udon noodles to the sauce and stir well to combine.
6. To serve, spoon into bowls and garnish each with fresh cilantro leaves, crushed peanuts, bean sprouts, lime wedges and chile to taste.

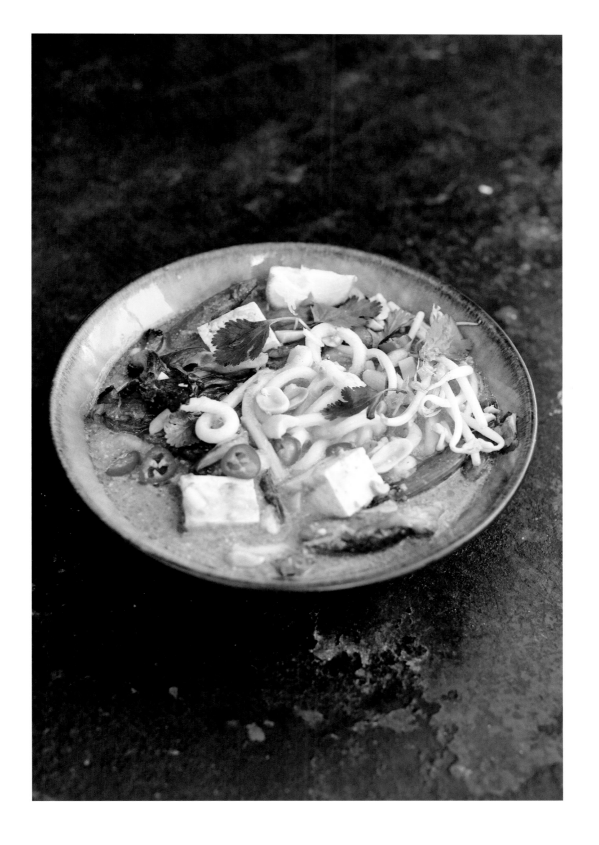

Chicken broth

50 CALORIES
PER ½ CUP

——

- Roast chicken carcass
  (see p. 230)
- Sea salt and black pepper

OPTIONAL EXTRAS
- Garlic cloves
- Onions, roughly chopped
- Celery stalks,
  roughly chopped
- Carrots, roughly chopped
- Sprigs of herbs (sage,
  oregano, thyme, rosemary,
  bay leaves)

Making bone broth from scratch means utilizing all the minerals found within the bones such as calcium, magnesium and phosphorus. This makes a much more nutritious base for stocks than a store-bought cube. I simply add the carcass from my roast to a big pot, cover with water and leave to simmer for a couple of hours. I might include other ingredients for additional flavoring, such as an onion, some garlic cloves or a few herbs – whatever I have on hand. The same applies to the bones: I've used a chicken carcass here, but you could use anything you have left over from a roast, such as turkey, lamb or beef. Just cook it for a good long time, keeping the water topped up and allowing the nutrients from the bones to permeate the broth for the full nutritional hit.

1. Place the chicken carcass in a large saucepan and cover with water so that it comes at least 1 inch above the bones.
2. Season with salt and pepper and bring to a boil, then reduce the heat and simmer for an hour. To intensify the flavor, you can continue to boil, topping up with water if needed.
3. When the broth has cooked to the desired strength, pour it through a sieve into a clean bowl or jar. Remove any skin and bones, retaining any bits of meat. (I always throw them back into the broth.)
4. Once made, the broth can be stored in the fridge for 3–4 days or frozen for future use (see tip below).

TIP
I like to freeze bone broth in ice-cube trays or small airtight plastic containers, so it is readily available to add to any number of dishes. I'll chuck a few cubes into Bolognese sauce, for instance, or a stir-fry or risotto.

Roasted Jerusalem artichokes and mixed roots

SERVES 4

————

165 CALORIES
PER SERVING

————

- 2 Jerusalem artichokes, peeled and cut into chunks
- 1 sweet potato (unpeeled), cut into chunks
- 4 parsnips (unpeeled), cut into chunks
- 1 turnip, peeled and cut into chunks
- 1 carrot, peeled and cut into chunks
- 1 tbsp raw coconut oil, melted
- 2 sprigs of rosemary
- Sea salt and black pepper

If you have never had Jerusalem artichokes, give this dish a try or cut them in half and roast them, either to eat like this or to mash up as an alternative to mashed potato. Once you've discovered them, they'll become a regular dish, I guarantee! Here I've roasted them with parsnips and sweet potato for a really tasty mix.

1. Preheat the oven to 400°F.
2. Place the Jerusalem artichokes, sweet potato and parsnips in a medium saucepan filled with water and parboil for 5 minutes.
3. Drain and place on a baking sheet or roasting pan. Add the remaining vegetables, drizzle with the melted coconut oil and toss together to coat.
4. Add the rosemary and seasoning and roast in the oven for 20 minutes or until crispy and brown.

Classic roast chicken
with turnips

SERVES 4—6

———

500 CALORIES
PER SERVING

———

FOR THE HERB BUTTER
- 4 tbsp (½ stick) butter, softened
- Leaves from 2 sprigs of rosemary, chopped
- Small bunch of fresh oregano, chopped
- Grated zest of 1 lemon, reserving the used lemon
- Sea salt and black pepper

- 1 whole chicken (about 4 lbs) with giblets
- 2 sprigs of rosemary
- 2 medium onions, halved
- 2 medium turnips, peeled and cut into quarters
- 2 sweet potatoes, peeled and cut into six
- 2 parsnips, peeled and cut into 1-inch pieces
- 2 large carrots, peeled and roughly chopped
- 1 tbsp olive oil
- 2 tbsp rice flour

I include turnips and other roots when I cook a classic roast chicken. It helps make the meal more nutritious and less calorific overall. A single serving of this nurturing dish offers a generous supply of the B vitamins riboflavin and niacin, which help to keep the skin well oxygenated and prevent dullness.

1. Preheat the oven to 400°F.
2. Place the butter in a bowl with the chopped herbs and lemon zest. Season with salt and pepper and mix so the butter is soft and everything is combined.
3. To prepare the chicken skin for stuffing, use a spoon to get between the skin and the meat. Start at the side of the cavity just above the legs and work toward the breastbone and up the back to create a large pocket.
4. Take some of the herb butter and push it into one side of the pocket you have created. Using your hands, smooth it inside and out over the top of the skin. Repeat this on the other side, then cut the skin of the legs and squash in any remaining butter mixture.
5. Fill the chicken cavity with the used lemon (cut in half) and the rosemary sprigs. Place the onion halves and giblets in a roasting pan and sit the chicken on top. Wrap the chicken in foil (covering the sides of the pan) and place in the oven to roast for 30 minutes.
6. Remove the foil and roast for another 30 minutes or until cooked through and golden brown on top.
7. Meanwhile, place the remaining vegetables in a large saucepan of water, bring to a boil and cook for 10 minutes. Drain, reserving the cooking water, and place back in the pan. Cover with a lid and give the vegetables a good shake to roughen the edges for a crispier finish. Add the vegetables to a separate roasting pan, drizzle with the oil and sprinkle with salt.
8. About 10 minutes before the chicken is cooked, place the vegetables in the oven to roast for 20 minutes.
9. Transfer the chicken to a board, cover in foil and leave to rest for 10 minutes. Drain off some of the fat from the pan, then place in a small saucepan over medium heat. Add the rice flour to the cooking juices and gradually stir in enough of the reserved vegetable-cooking liquid to make a smooth and pourable gravy.
10. Place pieces of carved chicken on plates and serve with the roasted vegetables and gravy.

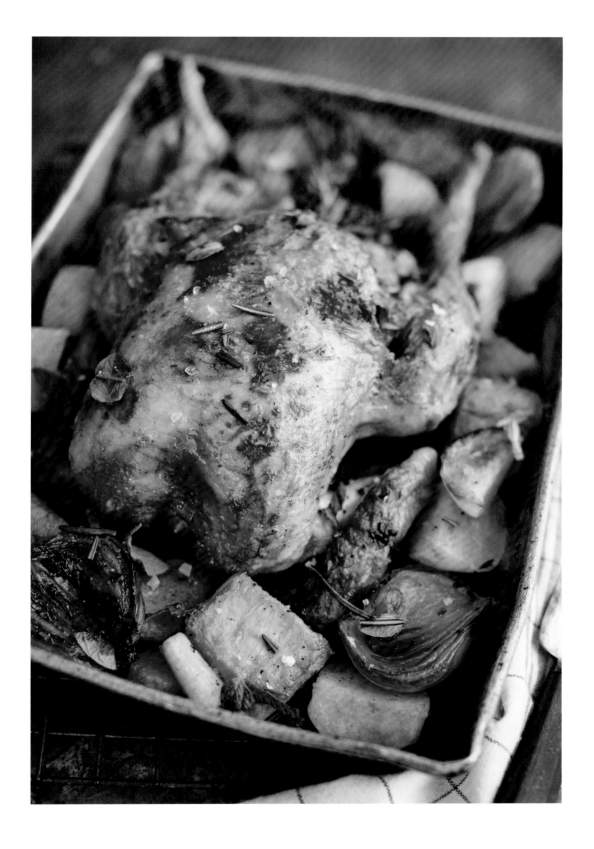

Gluten-free rhubarb crumble

SERVES 6

----

311 CALORIES
PER SERVING

- 6 tbsp rice flour
  (or other gluten-free flour)
- 3 tsp Stevia
- 1½ sticks butter, cut into
  cubes
- 2 handfuls of walnuts,
  crushed
- 10 sticks of rhubarb,
  cut into ½-inch pieces
- 1 apple, peeled,
  cored and chopped into
  bite-sized pieces
- Handful of dried
  cranberries
- Juice of ½ lemon

TO SERVE (OPTIONAL)
- Crème fraîche infused
  with a vanilla pod
  (halved and seeds removed)
- Vanilla ice cream

My mum used to make rhubarb crumble a lot; it always went down well. Whenever I make this gluten-free version, it's met with joyful approval from friends after a hearty meal in the depths of winter. The recipe is a twist on traditional crumble, using gluten-free flour with added walnuts for a dose of omega-3 fatty acids and antioxidants that are so essential for skin health.

1. Preheat the oven to 350°F.
2. Combine the flour and 2 teaspoons of the Stevia in a mixing bowl. Using your fingertips, rub in the butter until the mixture is crumbly in texture. Add the walnuts and set aside.
3. Place the rhubarb, apple and cranberries in a large saucepan with 2 tablespoons of water and the rest of the Stevia. Cook down over medium heat for 10–15 minutes or until the fruit is plump, soft and juicy but still holding its shape.
4. Add the lemon juice to the fruit mixture and stir to combine.
5. Place the cooked fruit in a small ovenproof dish and top with the crumble mixture. Bake in the oven for 20 minutes or until browned on top, and serve with vanilla-infused crème fraîche or ice cream, if you wish.

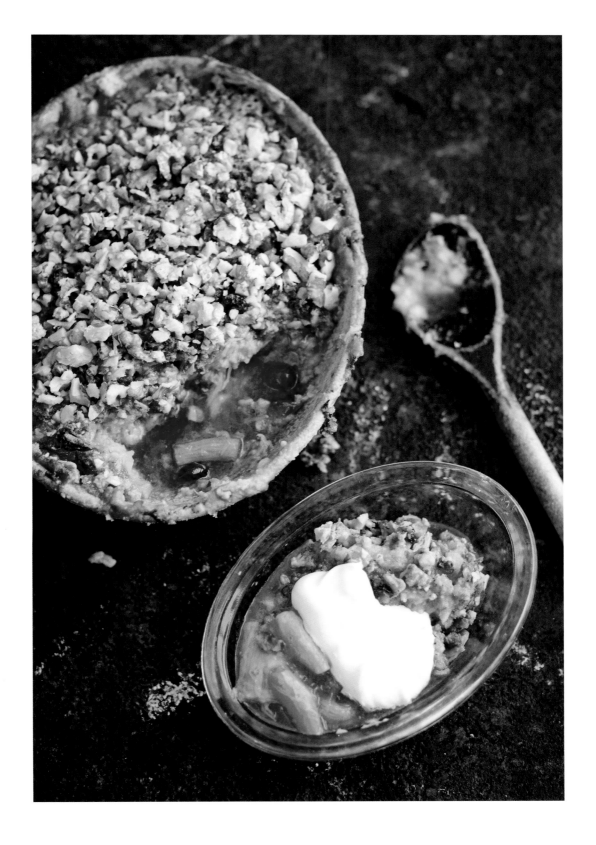

Flourless orange and almond cake

SERVES 8

―――

271 CALORIES
PER SERVING

―――

- 2 oranges
- Butter or coconut oil, for greasing
- 3 eggs
- 1 cup superfine sugar
- 10 oz ground almonds
- 1 tsp baking powder
- 1 tbsp chopped pistachios, for sprinkling

This is a great, no-nonsense dessert for the colder months, and it's so easy! Do be aware, it does contain a lot of sugar, so it's not something for every day – especially if you have skin problems – but lovely for a special treat. The zesty orange flavor complements the moist, slightly nutty texture of the sponge, which has the advantage of being gluten-free. A good alternative to standard wheat flour, ground almonds contain all the nutrients of the whole nut, including vitamin E, which is important for healthy skin.

1. Place the oranges in a medium saucepan and cover with cold water. Bring to a boil, then reduce the heat and cook for 1 hour or until tender. Transfer to a food processor and blend until smooth.
2. Preheat the oven to 400°F, then grease a 9-inch-diameter cake pan with a little butter or coconut oil and line the base with parchment paper.
3. Place the eggs and sugar in a mixing bowl and, using an electric beater, whisk until thick and pale. Add the puréed oranges, ground almonds and baking powder, and gently fold in to combine.
4. Pour the cake batter into the prepared pan and bake for 1 hour or until springy to the touch. Leave in the pan to cool for about 5 minutes before transferring to a wire rack to finish cooling. Sprinkle with the pistachios before slicing to serve.

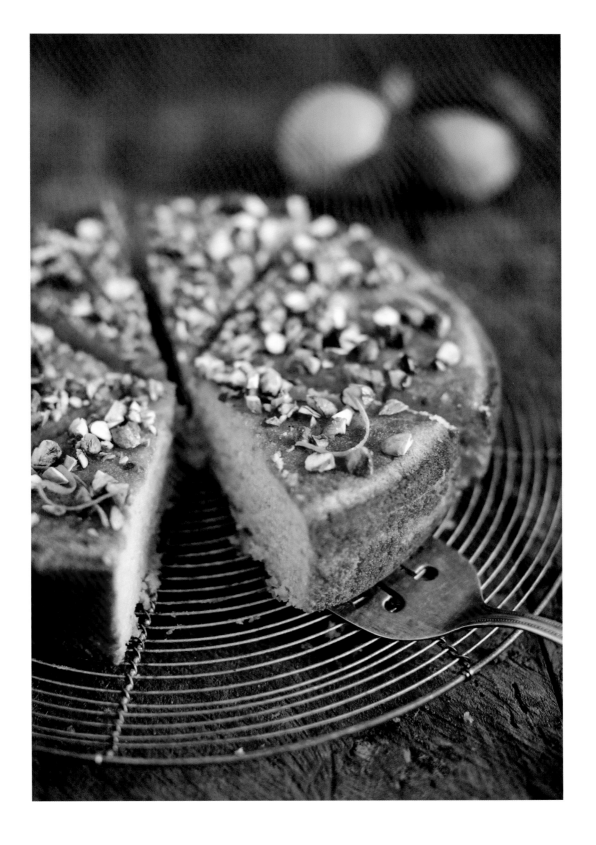

Rosemary tea

SERVES 4

‒‒‒‒

8 CALORIES
PER CUP

‒‒‒‒

- 2–3 sprigs of rosemary
- 4 tsp molasses, to serve
(optional)

This helps to calm my digestive system while working to keep my skin looking youthful. This caffeine-free tea is a delicious way to keep you hydrated – a plus both for your digestion and your skin.

1. Place the sprigs in a teapot and fill with boiling water, then pour into teacups to serve. Alternatively, strip the leaves from the rosemary sprigs, then chop them up and place in a tea strainer. Place the strainer over a teacup and pour over boiling water before filling the remaining three cups in the same way.
2. Serve each cupful with a teaspoon of molasses, if you like.

Coconut kefir

SERVES 4

‒‒‒‒

30 CALORIES
PER SERVING

‒‒‒‒

- Starter sachet of
kefir grains
- 5 cups coconut water

You can use milk, but I like to make this using coconut water. I drink it before breakfast or bed, giving it time to work in the gut without any food. Sachets are easily obtainable online.

1. Empty the sachet into a bowl and add coconut water to cover. Stir to a paste until the lumps have dissolved.
2. Pour in more liquid and gently stir until smooth, using the back of a spoon to break up any lumps.
3. Gradually add more coconut water (until about half full) and continue stirring for 5–10 minutes. It is important that the culture is mixed thoroughly (see tip below).
4. Pour into a jar and add the remaining coconut water, then mix for 10 minutes, so that the culture is evenly distributed. This is vital to ensure even fermentation.
5. Cover and leave somewhere warm to ferment – between 18 and 30 hours. Don't stir during this time. The finished mix will look separated, with a frothy head and fizzy taste. Stir and serve. Store in the fridge for 4 days.

TIP
- For step 3, you can pour the mixture into a food processor and blend on a slow speed for 5–10 minutes. Pour in the remaining coconut water (step 4) and blend for 10 minutes.

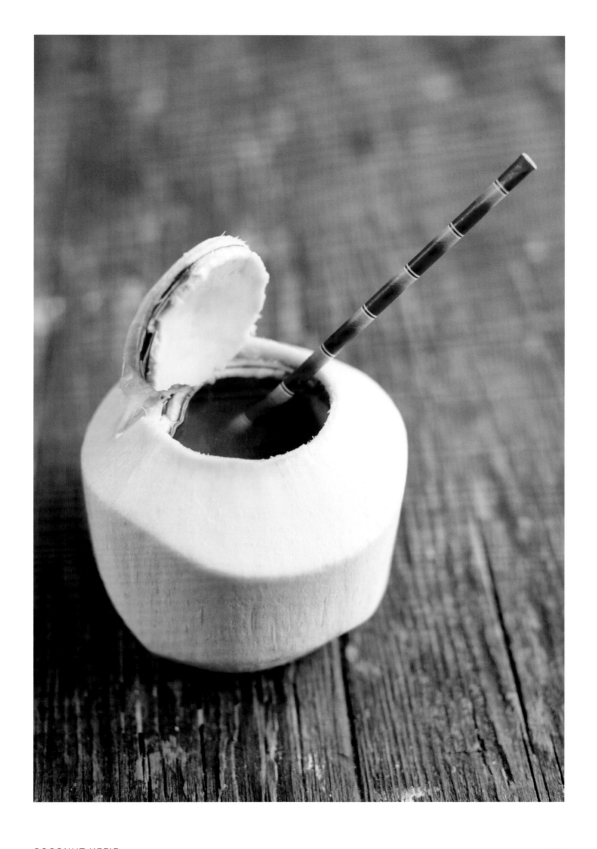

COCONUT KEFIR

Mulled natural wine

- 3 oranges, juiced and peel cut into strips
- 1 lemon, peel cut into strips
- 1 lime, peel cut into strips
- 2 tbsp honey
- 2–4 cloves
- 1 cinnamon stick
- 2 bay leaves
- 1 tsp grated nutmeg
- 1 vanilla pod, halved and seeded
- 2 (750ml) bottles of natural red wine
- 2 star anise

As a special festive treat, is there anything better than a glass of mulled wine? I love the spicy aroma of the red wine warming in a pan on the burner – perfect for a chilly winter evening to enjoy with friends.

1. Place the cut peel from all the citrus fruit in a large saucepan and add the honey, cloves, cinnamon stick, bay leaves and nutmeg.
2. Throw in the halved vanilla pod and the orange juice and pour in just enough wine to cover all the ingredients.
3. Bring to a simmer to dissolve the honey, then increase the heat and boil for 5 minutes or until the mixture has thickened to a syrup-like consistency.
4. Add the star anise, followed by the rest of the wine. Increase the heat to allow the mixture to warm through for a few minutes, and then serve.

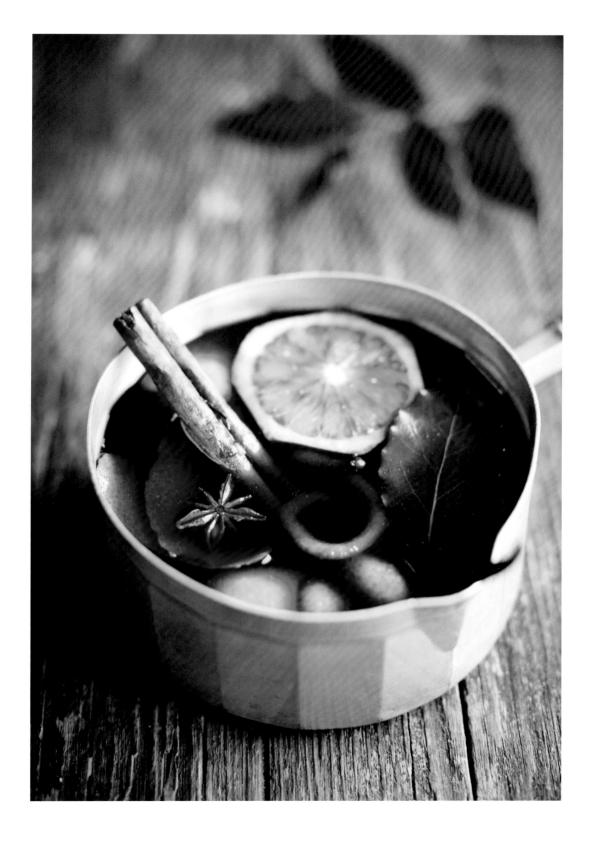

beauty tips

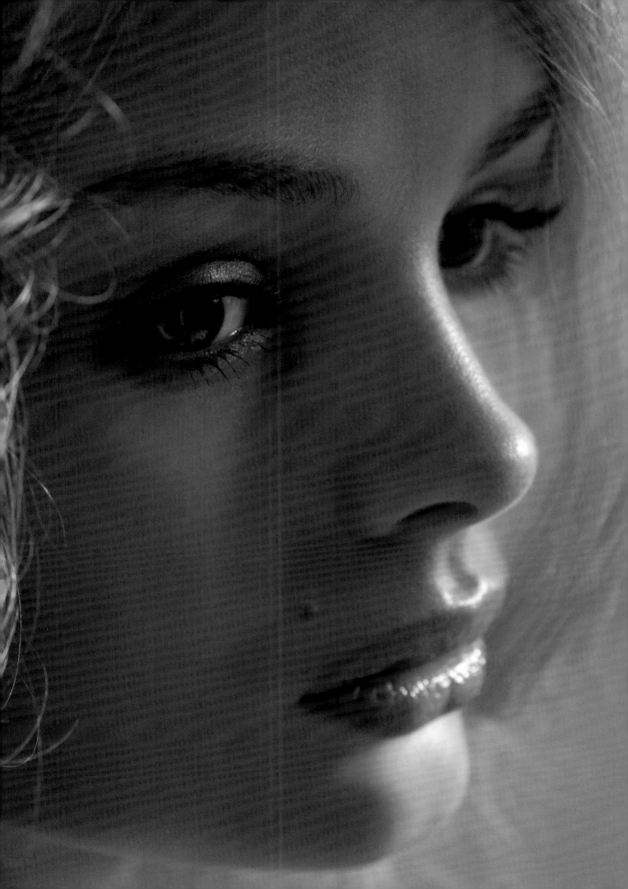

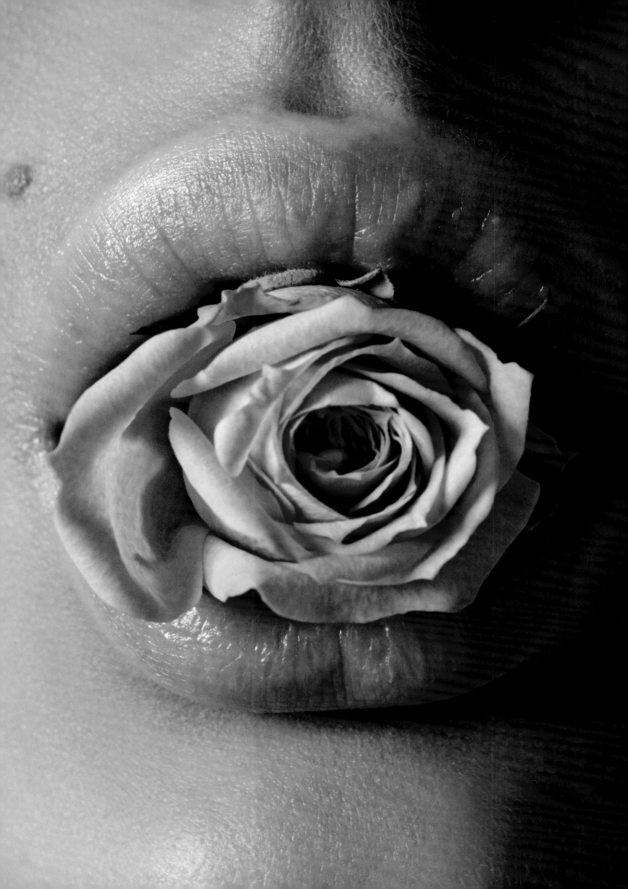

Rosewater toner

Homemade rosewater is genius. A multi-tasking gem, it not only nourishes, hydrates and balances, but it smells incredible and has antibacterial properties. Opt for organic roses when possible; commercial varieties are heavily sprayed with chemicals.

- 1 mug of rose petals, fresh or dried
- 2 mugs of boiling mineral water
- 1 spray bottle and a piece of muslin or cheesecloth

1. Place the petals in a heat-resistant bowl and add the boiling water, then cover with a lid. Leave to infuse for 30 minutes.
2. Strain into the bottle. Discard the petals.
3. Soak a cotton pad in the rosewater and dab on your face as a toner after cleansing and before applying moisturizer. To revive tired or puffy eyes, place a soaked cotton pad over each eye and leave on for a couple of minutes.
4. Store in the fridge for 2–3 weeks.

HERBAL TONERS

- Substitute the roses with lavender flowers or fresh herbs (rosemary, mint).
- I like to spray a washcloth with toner and then pop it in a freezer bag in the fridge to use after a workout or on a hot day.

Magnesium foot scrub

Named after the spring in Surrey where the minerals were first discovered, Epsom salts (chemically known as magnesium sulfate) provide countless benefits to health, both inside and out. I use the salts in a foot scrub. This has the dual action of smoothing rough skin and allowing the body to absorb the much-needed magnesium – a mineral that's important for maintaining healthy bones and detoxifying the body but which many people are deficient in. I add peppermint oil. Remember to clean your feet first! This makes 1–2 scrubs, so store any extra in an airtight jar. Use no more than twice a week.

- 1 teacup or mug of Epsom salts
- ¼ teacup or mug of almond oil
- 10–15 drops of essential oil

1. In a bowl, mix all the ingredients and add essential oil – I like it quite gritty.
2. To apply, scoop up a handful of the mixture and massage it into the top and sole of each foot, including the ankle. Leave on for 5 minutes before washing off in the shower. Alternatively, add a scoop of the mixture to a footbath and soak your feet in it for a few minutes.

EPSOM SALT BATH

An Epsom salt bath after exercise helps get rid of the lactic acid build-up that can make muscles sore. Add 2 handfuls of salts and 2–4 drops of essential oil to your bath and enjoy!

Calming lavender mist

I always use lavender mist when I'm prepping a model's skin. It soothes the skin, due to its anti-inflammatory properties, and calms everyone (including me!). I remove it with a tissue before moisturizing. I've included witch hazel, which treats blemishes, but leave out otherwise as it can be drying.

- ½ cup mineral water
- 1 tsp witch hazel (optional)
- 5 drops of lavender essential oil (preferably organic)
- 1 spray bottle

1. Pour it all into the bottle and shake.
2. Spray directly after cleansing and before moisturizing or whenever your skin feels oily or needs a pick-me-up. It will keep well in the fridge for up to 6 months.

Coconut oil cleanser

The antibacterial properties of raw coconut oil make it very useful as a topical treatment for the skin, helping to cleanse and neutralize toxins. It's great for a range of skin problems, from breakouts, red blotchy or dry patches to mild acne. I use it as a hand moisturizer, too. Simply apply as a hand cream.

- 1 tsp raw coconut oil

1. Gently massage your face with the oil.
2. Wait 20 seconds and remove with a warm, wet cloth.

Spirulina face mask

Packed with antioxidants, this restores a healthy glow and protects the skin from the aging effects of airborne pollutants.

- 1–2 tsp spirulina powder
- 1 tsp of raw coconut oil (optional)
- 1–2 teaspoons of mineral water

1. Mix the ingredients into a smooth paste.
2. Apply and leave for 5–10 minutes. Use a foundation brush. Wash off in the shower using a washcloth.

Inhalation

Essential oils are great for so many reasons.

DECONGESTANT

Add 5–10 drops of oil (such as eucalyptus or tea tree) to a bowl of steaming water. Place a towel over your head and bowl and inhale for 5–10 minutes. Repeat 2–3 times a day.

FACIAL STEAM

Add one drop of chamomile, juniper, lavender and petitgrain oils to steaming water.

TREATMENT FOR ACNE

Combine equal parts of chickweed, elderflower and marigold oils. Add 5–10 drops of the mix to steaming water. Steam for 5–10 minutes.

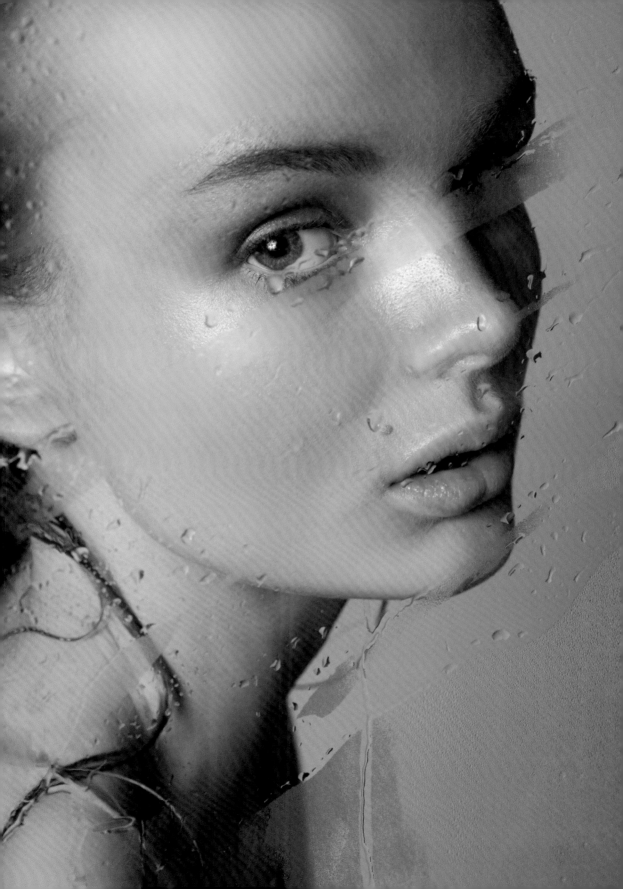

Non-negotiable skincare routine

NIGHT

- Just before you go to bed, wash your face with a gentle neutral cleanser, rinse off, then put on a toner with a cotton pad or spray. Apply a moisturizer and eye cream.
- Once or twice a week, treat your face with an oil or night cream.
- Once a week, apply a face mask.
- Once a week or less you should exfoliate, but this is really down to personal preference.

MORNING

- First thing, wash your face with cold water and then use a toner.
- Apply moisturizer and an eye cream.

NOTE If any products sting when applied to your skin, they are not right for you. Opt for something designed for sensitive skin.

"Wendy was a pioneer of the 'natural' look long before it became a current obsession – one of the very first makeup artists to realize that beautiful skin comes from the inside. And she practices what she preaches, encouraging models to eat healthily."
— **Kathy Phillips,** beauty director, Condé Nast International

Cleansers

There are several different types of cleanser: foaming, cleansing wash, cream or oil. You need to choose what feels right for you. It is really about how your skin feels afterward. If you're a younger person and your skin produces quite a lot of oil, a cleansing wash can be best. As you get older, a cream or an oil may be better for you. Opt for a good, neutral cleanser and just cleanse at the end of the day right before you go to bed. Try to avoid perfumed cleansers, as they won't be made from natural ingredients and you may have a reaction if you have sensitive skin. If your skin feels really tight this is not right for you because you have removed too much of the natural oil, causing the pores to overproduce oil and taking you back to square one!

The reasons for cleansing only at night are:

- To remove all the dirt from airborne pollutants you will have come into contact with during the day.
- To leave your skin clean to repair itself.
- If you cleanse again in the morning you will remove the natural oils that are your skin's natural balance and it may cause your skin to overproduce oil.

Toners

You need to use a good toner with not too much alcohol in it; rosewater makes an excellent one (see p. 243). I use a reviving one in the morning for closing my pores, and a gentler, less astringent toner in the evening to remove any cleanser still left on and restore a nice balance. You can use quite a milky toner at night for added nourishment.

Moisturizers

A moisturizer is a must-have – needed to hydrate and protect your skin against the elements. It should change with the seasons. When the weather's warm, opt for lighter; in the colder months, go for heavier. This is common sense – just as you switch from lighter to heavier clothing during the year.

Exfoliation

Exfoliation – the removing of dead skin cells – is an essential part of luminous-looking skin: your complexion can't look fresh when it's congested with dull, dead cells. Depending on your skin type, you can opt for a home exfoliator (something with gritty bits in it) or a chemical/fruit acid exfoliator. It's important to choose the right formula for your skin type, so get advice from a beauty therapist/dermatologist – and don't overdo it. I hardly ever exfoliate – only once every couple of weeks or when I need a reboot, in which case I'd see a specialist. People tend to exfoliate too much and then are surprised that their skin is sensitive and dry or too oily. No wonder – you just removed all the natural oils from your face!

Night oils

Maybe once a week, I put on a night oil. These oils penetrate deeper than a moisturizer. People think it will make their skin greasy and trigger an outbreak, but if your skin is clean, there's no reason why you would get spots. If you're putting oil on dirty skin, then you skipped step one of my "Non-negotiable Skincare Routine," so start over!

Face masks

Face masks are brilliant for giving your skin a lift and pulling out any dirt that may have built up, causing congestion. I use a face mask once every 1–2 weeks depending on time – a cleansing one if my skin's a bit oily, or a more hydrating one if it's feeling dry. There are lots of different types: clay masks to draw out all the toxins and impurities – good if you have problem or oily skin; cream masks that brighten and hydrate; ones to encourage better circulation in the face. It depends very much on your individual needs. After a long flight, I like to use a hydrating paper mask, for instance, to help restore moisture as the recycled air in the pressurized cabin can dry out the skin.

Facial massage

On set it's part of my job to make an instant assessment of a model's skin. One of the ways I do this is through facial massage, which I perform with cream. I cleanse the face before applying makeup. It stimulates blood flow and lymph drainage, as well as helping remove dead skin. You can include this technique in your own daily regimen. Use a cream cleanser or facial cleansing oil and massage it gently into the skin with your fingertips. This clears extra fluid from the face, giving it more definition. Areas to focus on include the sinus points along the nasal passageways, the temples, under the cheekbones and along the jawline. It helps to release built-up tension, making your face look more relaxed. See my website for a short video demonstration (wendyrowe.com).

Go to wendyrowe.com for the most up-to-date skincare brand recommendations.

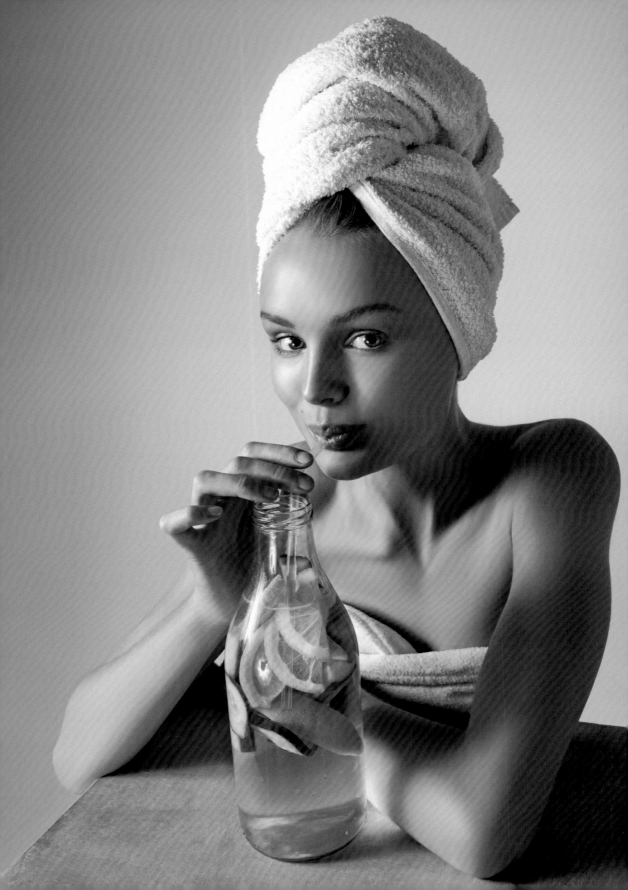

Water is essential – integral to the function of every organ. Getting enough should be the first step in treating your skin from within; there is literally no way for the skin to glow without proper hydration. When you don't take in enough water, your blood draws water from the skin cells, leading to a dull and lifeless complexion. This dehydration makes the skin less elastic and less able to defend itself, making it more prone to wrinkling over time.

I often deal with dehydrated skin in my work – dry lips and a flaky surface are a giveaway. People always say how they find water boring and so opt for sugary drinks or coffee. This not only ages the skin by killing collagen, but it triggers blood-sugar and doesn't rehydrate.

Infusions

If you're not keen on pure water, then adding flavorsome extras makes a great alternative.

CUCUMBER AND MINT

Cut half a cucumber into slices and place in a pitcher. Squeeze the juice of a lemon into the pitcher, then slice up a second lemon and throw it in, too. Add a few sprigs of mint and pour water over. Add some ice and serve.

HERBAL

Place 1 teaspoonful of dried herbs into a teapot and add boiling water. Leave to stand for 10 minutes before straining or transfer to a pitcher and add ice. Always use good-quality herbs, preferably organic, from a health-food store. If using fresh herbs, finely chop and use 2 teaspoons per pot.

Acne

Sufferers know better than anyone the distress "angry" skin brings. There's no one cause, it can be a sign that something is wrong at a deeper level. The skin produces too much sebum (natural oils secreted by the sebaceous glands), causing congestion and subsequent infection. The pores become filled with the excess sebum, which traps dead skin cells and – along with overproduction of a protein called keratin – forms a plug. This stops the sebum exiting the pore and causes a build-up of bacteria. Hormones can play a big part, such as during puberty (with the increase in testosterone) or pregnancy, if you're taking birth control pills or if you're suffering from polycystic ovarian syndrome (PCOS). It's well worth having a chat with your doctor or specialist.

Increasingly we're learning that diet is hugely important, with sugar, gluten and dairy being the main offenders. So it's worth cutting out the potential culprits, and observing the changes through a process of elimination. There are foods that are said to fight acne – sweet potatoes, Brazil nuts, pumpkin seeds and red peppers – thanks to their high levels of zinc, selenium, essential fatty acids, vitamin A and beta-carotene. You also need to keep your skin cleansed and hydrated. I had bad skin as a teenager. I would take 1,000mg of time-release vitamin C supplements daily; use a gentle foaming cleanser (see p. 246); and dab a little skin antiseptic on the problem areas at night. What will help (but is a pain in the ass!) is using disposable towels and changing your pillowcase daily. And don't touch your face, as you don't want to spread the bacteria! This advice is great for teenagers too. Manuka honey is useful for acne sufferers (see p. 262).

Rosacea

Another maddening condition, this begins with a subtle redness to the face which, if left untreated, usually worsens. It can include small spots or in advance cases, lobules on the skin, and a tendency to flush. Like many skin conditions, there's plenty of debate about what causes it, but I believe it's a symptom of wider inflammation in the body. If your diet is full of acid-forming foods, for instance – especially alcohol, sugar, dairy and gluten – you may be more susceptible. And if you have more sensitive or fine skin, you're more likely to suffer from a light form of it, though that's all down to the genes, unfortunately.

A connection has been suggested between the gut and rosacea and taking a probiotic – an organic one with no sugar – may help. Omit foods that are acid-forming.

Rosacea is a temperamental condition and responds to a simple diet, rich in whole foods, and a careful skincare regimen. Dermatologists recommend avoiding perfumed skincare products. If hypoallergenic skincare products don't work, try organic. Drinking alcohol does not help.

Eczema

Thought to be linked to allergic disease, eczema sits in the same category as asthma and hay fever. And like those conditions, it normally starts when you're a child. A trigger seems to set off the condition, and the immune system goes into attack mode, leaving the skin dry, red and itchy. It's this itching sensation, which is caused by the release of histamine stimulating the nerve endings, that drives sufferers up the wall.

As in all skin conditions, stress is a common culprit. Certain foods and environmental factors can cause a flare-up, too, so try cutting out the foods you suspect might be a trigger. I'd recommend seeing a nutritionist or naturopath. Foods that fight eczema include those rich in zinc, essential fatty acids, B-complex vitamins or beta-carotene.

Psoriasis

Characterized by patches of red and scaly skin, it is a relatively common skin condition and varies in severity. It seems to be caused by too-rapid cell turnover, with increased shedding of skin cells. The new skin doesn't have time to settle, leaving it itchy and irritated. It's best to see your doctor, and you'll probably be referred to a dermatologist, usually for a cream or ointment but this is a band aid, not a solution. See a naturopath.

Foods rich in fatty acids will help keep the inflammation at bay. Opting, too, for foods rich in B-complex vitamins is excellent for regulating the cell turnover and fighting inflammation. Symptoms can be alleviated by sunshine and swimming in the sea – a great excuse to take a holiday! Stress can play a part (another reason to take a break). Evening primrose oil may be beneficial: take a 500mg capsule daily for 2–3 months.

TAILORING YOUR SKINCARE

———

Below are a few guidelines on skin types. Everyone's complexion is unique, often a combination rather than just one type, so a one-size-fits-all approach to skincare simply won't work. These are just a few pointers, feel free to mix and match; if something doesn't feel good, you can just wipe it off.

Oily skin

If you have oily skin, it's good in a way because the oilier the skin, the fewer lines you'll get. On the other hand, if your body overproduces oil, it can make you prone to getting pimples.

_____

SELF-HELP TIPS

- Apply a clay mask once a week – this draws quite a lot of the sebum (oil) and toxins out of the skin.
- Use a mattifying moisturizer to help reduce shine.
- Don't overload with creams.
- Don't wear makeup all the time.
- Try using an oil-control foundation.
- Find a good routine for yourself; a foaming cleanser may be better than an oil cleanser, for instance.
- Try to do a scrub once a week, as you might find you have a build-up of dead skin which can lead to the overproduction of sebum.
- Eat tomatoes as they are good for targeting excess sebum production.
- Avoid eating deep-fried food.
- Make sure you exercise – sweating is great for clearing the pores.

Mature skin

Collagen is what keeps the face full and youthful, but we stop producing it after the age of 25. As we grow older, the connective tissue starts to loosen and the elasticity reduces, causing the face to droop. There's no miracle cream that will reverse the signs of aging; you can only try to slow down the process. Eating a healthy diet, full of skin-benefiting foods, should be the first step, along with exercise and a good skincare routine (see p. 246). I always think it's best to nurture what you've got – allow your face to have character as it's much more attractive than too much botox and fillers that erase the face you were born with, even if it's changed over time. But for very fine lines, listen, a bit of baby botox is fine!

_____

SELF-HELP TIPS

- Use a cream cleanser, rosewater and a cream moisturizer, but bear in mind that no cream will ever erase lines.
- Have a facial on a regular basis.
- To keep the elasticity in the skin, try a collagen drink like Skinade.
- Make sure you take vitamin K2 and calcium supplements, as they are really good for the bones, and these nutrients tend to deplete as you get older.
- Make sure you take iron tablets.
- For unwanted pigmentation, take a selenium supplement (preferably organic) to treat it from within.
- For dark circles under the eyes, take a tablespoon of molasses every day.

Professional treatment

- If you really want to eradicate lines, you could try a strong skin peel. This has to be done by a recommended doctor or dermatologist, not by a beautician.
- Botox is an option. It will get rid of lines, but it is a toxin, so it's better to have less than too much. It has to be done by a specialist and not a beautician.
- Mesotherapy – injections of collagen and other nutrients via ultra-fine needles – can restore a glow and help with unwanted pigmentation. This has to be done by a specialist.

"Wendy is a ball of creative, loving and energetic fire. She always has a fresh take on a look that pays off and is never shy of an impromptu boogie. Wendy takes me to Neverland."— **Suki Waterhouse**, actress and model

Teenage skincare basics

Being a teenager is hard. Raging hormones, school work, a social life and your skin can go a bit haywire – just at the time you don't have the confidence to deal with it. I do understand that you're living by your parents' rules: you want to be independent but you have no money to buy the things that you think you need, and this all adds to the frustration. My advice is to be nice to your parents and they might buy you some skincare products! Or, get a job and buy your own! And start to look after your skin, too. It will pay dividends in the long run. Why do you think models look so good? They take care of their skin, through watching what they eat and following a good skincare routine. A lot of the models I work with are very young, but you can tell the ones who have learned to look after their skin from the ones who haven't. With a head start like this, you'll look and feel great and can thank me when you get older.

In addition to the guidelines listed in my "Non-negotiable Skincare Routine" (see p. 246), here are a few basics. They work wonders, I promise – they certainly did for me when I was younger and had bad skin – plus they're super cheap:

SELF-HELP TIPS

- Take a 1,000mg time-release vitamin C capsule daily.
- Use a foaming cleanser at night.
- If you have acne, dab a little skin antiseptic onto affected areas at night.
- Use a really light moisturizing lotion.
- Use a simple lavender mist (see p. 244) as a toner morning and night.
- Acne might be an issue (see p. 249).

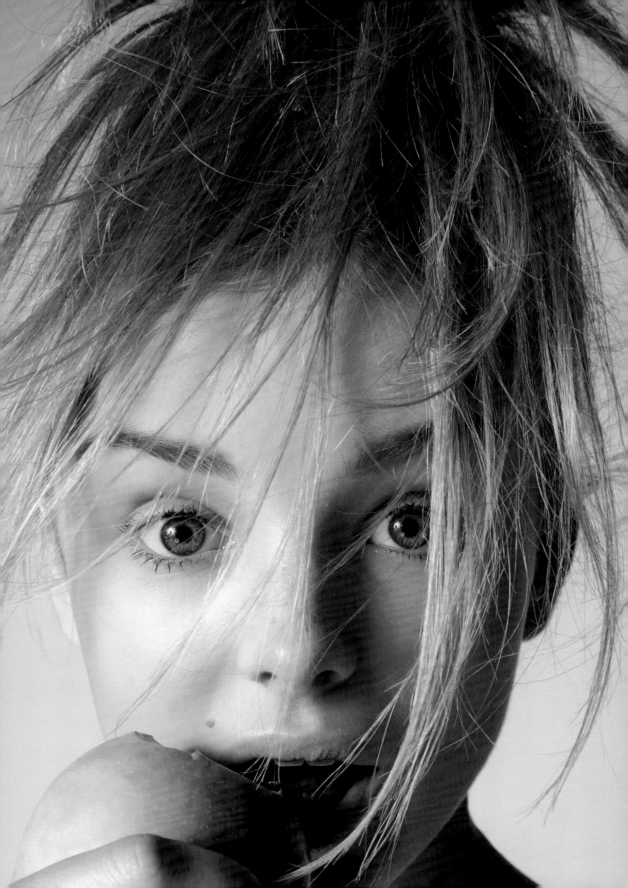

SUNCARE

Navigating the maze of suncare information out there can be daunting, with conflicting information about the best way to protect your skin from harmful – and aging – UV rays and unwanted pigmentation. One thing most people agree on is that excess sun exposure can harm and prematurely age your skin, and can cause skin cancers, too. I make sure I take protection from the sun really seriously, but I also enjoy being in it and soaking up the essential vitamin D it provides. Here's what I've learned on the subject so far.

UVA AND UVB RAYS

Short-wave ultraviolet (UV B) rays cause burning while long-wave (UV A) rays, which penetrate the skin more deeply, are the ones responsible for aging and sun damage that you will see years down the line – including damage to the skin's elastin and collagen, plus pigmentation and enlargement of blood vessels. A good-quality, broad-spectrum sunscreen protects against both.

"Wendy is by far one of the most forward, fun and fast makeup artists I know. She knows exactly what she wants and applies all skincare and foundations in a massage-like way – it is always a blessing being in her chair." — **Toni Garrn,** model

TYPES OF SUNSCREEN

There are two ways to protect skin from burning and damage: either "physical" sunscreens (comprising zinc oxide or titanium dioxide), which work to physically block the sun, or the "chemical" type (containing encamsule and triazine), which act as a filter to absorb or scatter the sun's rays. While the chemical types aren't visible on the skin and tend to be much lighter, most experts recommend a physical sunscreen as they offer protection against all UV rays and don't irritate sensitive skin.

SPF NUMBER

In case you didn't know, SPF stands for "sun protection factor." Although it might be confusing, the numbers don't refer to how long you can stay in the sun, but to the amount of UV protection the product offers. People often – wrongly – believe that by choosing a lower SPF they'll tan more quickly, but this increases the risk of burning and long-term skin damage – and you're more likely to get an uneven tan and your skin will peel as a result because it's burned. It's better to tan slowly. Start with a high SPF, applied properly, and as your skin builds a tan you can graduate to a cream with a lower SPF; this will help it last longer, too. It's important to apply sunscreen properly – the benchmark is a good 15 teaspoons for the whole body – and to reapply every 2 hours, or straight after a swim or sweaty activity. I love to lie in the shade on holiday – I find you get just as brown but don't burn. Some of my friends get annoyed that I end up with a better, more even tan and I didn't try as hard. Trust me, it works!

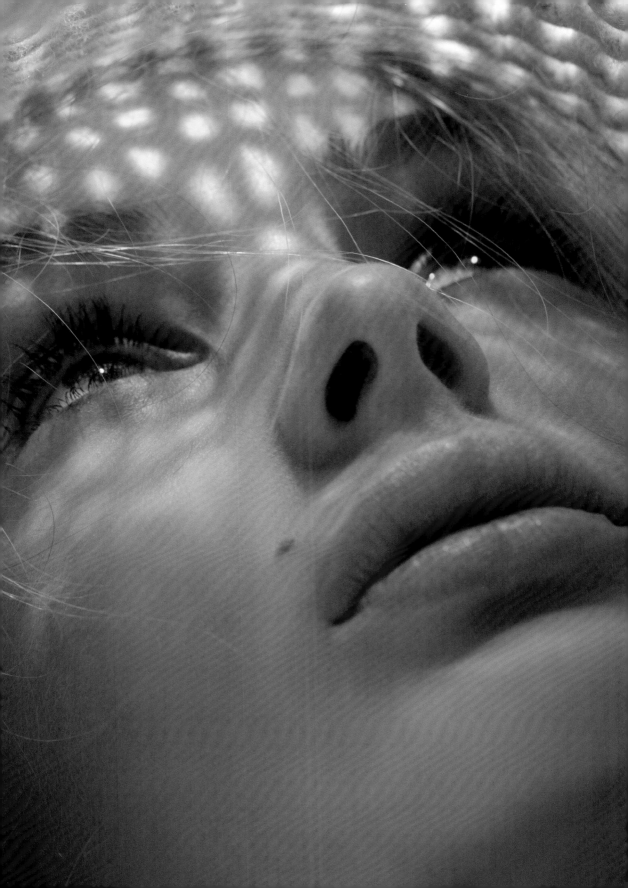

HEALING HERBS
AND SPICES

—

Nature's pharmacy

Modern medicines can be based on the oldest natural treatments known to humankind, with herbs and spices providing some of the most powerful resources in the search for radiant skin. Whether used topically, taken orally or added to cooking, these are my favorite skin-boosting ingredients from nature's pharmacy.

ALOE VERA

The ancient Egyptians called aloe vera the "plant of immortality" due to its ability to heal the skin, stimulate new cell growth and reduce redness. Helpful in the treatment of chronic skin disorders like acne, psoriasis and eczema, it's best used in its pure form, straight from the plant. It can be very effective for reducing scarring. My best friend who had chickenpox as an adult used to scoop the gel from an aloe vera leaf and apply it straight onto the skin every night, which completely eliminated the scars – which were really bad! Choose an organic, high-quality, filtered version of the juice to reap the rewards for your skin. Its ability to calm internal inflammation for a clearer, brighter-looking complexion. The fresh whole leaf is also delicious chopped and mixed with slices of fresh cucumber and mint leaves as a salad. Applied topically it can also be used to treat burns, including sunburn. — *Use in the form of juice, capsules, gel or cream*

BASIL

Basil has been used throughout history as a treatment for aging skin. The herb is a rich source of antioxidants and other nutrients that are essential for healthy skin. Vitamin A, in particular, is helpful in the treatment of acne. Simply including fresh basil in your diet will help your complexion, especially if you eat it raw. I love to have a pot growing on the windowsill. — *Use in the form of the fresh herb*

BURDOCK ROOT

An excellent anti-inflammatory, the root has been used for hundreds of years in treating all forms of chronic skin problems, including acne and eczema. Rich in fatty acids, burdock stimulates blood flow, boosting the circulation and helping to detoxify the body. I infuse a thumb-sized amount of the dried root (buy from any good health-food store) in a cup of boiling water, with a teaspoon of honey, for a homemade tea. As an oil extract, burdock can be applied directly to the skin. — *Use in the form of the dried root, tea, capsules or oil*

CALENDULA

Calendula cream is easy to find in a health-food store. Great for treating "angry" or dry skin conditions like psoriasis and dermatitis, it's something to always keep in your medicine cabinet – an all-purpose healing cream. Known for its calming properties, the plant extract helps soothe irritated or inflamed skin and is therefore perfect for treating acne, eczema and skin rashes. — *Use in the form of a cream, oil, powder or tea*

CAYENNE PEPPER

Loaded with antioxidants, cayenne pepper is known for its ability to treat acne by increasing blood flow to the skin. Packed with vitamins A and C, cayenne helps prevent the breakdown of collagen, while the capsaicin (a phytochemical) acts as an internal sunscreen to shield skin from UV damage. It's tasty and excellent for getting the blood flowing. I find that a sprinkling in a morning juice with lemon makes a great energy kick-start for the day. A big believer in its skin-benefiting powers. — *Use in the form of the ground spice*

CHAMOMILE

A powerful anti-inflammatory, chamomile reduces redness and swelling and has a soothing and calming effect on troubled skin. Used for thousands of years as a medicinal treatment, it contains the phytochemical azulene, which helps clean the pores of impurities and reduces puffiness. I love steeping a tablespoon of dried flowerheads in a cup of hot water after a long shoot. It helps me to wind down and sleep soundly. Chamomile is traditionally used in skincare formulas for its calming properties, so if aggravated skin is your issue, look out for chamomile extract in the ingredients. — *Use in the form of dried flowerheads, tea, cream or ointment*

CINNAMON

Cinnamon is such a valuable spice to have in your cupboard. Packed with antioxidants, it helps to address free-radical damage to the body caused by factors such as too much sun, which can prematurely age the skin. It's also great to use when you're trying to cut down on refined sugar, helping to satisfy sweet cravings without the downside of blood-sugar spikes and resulting breakouts. I sprinkle it in powdered form on porridge or in desserts and I include a cinnamon stick in a whole range of savory dishes or a tea. Chai teas, which are full of cinnamon, make a great alternative to coffee. — *Use in the form of the whole or ground spice*

CLOVE

Full of skin-friendly minerals (including calcium, iron and magnesium) and vitamins (C, E and K), clove is also a natural anesthetic and hence excellent in the battle against acne, helping to treat blackheads, whiteheads and pimples. Oil of clove is incredible for clearing skin, though it has to be used mixed with a carrier oil like almond oil to avoid irritation. I use it in a ratio of 1:10 (one part clove oil to ten parts almond oil), then apply it directly to a pimple and leave to dry it out overnight. Seriously effective. — *Use in the form of whole/ground spice or oil*

COMFREY

Rich in allantoin, a phytochemical that protects the skin and promotes cell growth, comfrey is a powerful healing herb that can be used to help "knit" cells together in damaged skin. It's best applied topically in the form of an ointment, although it can be taken as a leaf tea for a general health tonic. — *Use in the form of an ointment, oil or tea*

CUMIN

The prophet Muhammad apparently prized black cumin as "a remedy for every illness except death" and the seeds have been used for centuries to help improve the condition of hair, nails and skin. Packed with nutrients – essential fatty acids, protein, flavonoids, vitamins A, B and C and calcium, potassium, magnesium and zinc – cumin helps the skin to heal itself. It's therefore great for using in the treatment of conditions like acne, rosacea and irregular pigmentation. Using cumin in your cooking is a great way to get a dose and the spice is integral to curries, which I love. Something like a simple dhal is a great way to get cumin seeds into the diet, helping both to clear the skin and add flavor. — *Use in the form of whole or ground spice*

DANDELION

It's easy to view dandelions as nothing more than a troublesome weed, but actually they're a powerful healing herb. Packed with vitamins A, B, C and D, it promotes a clear complexion and helps the body eliminate unwanted skin bacteria. I put a handful of the leaves in a cup of hot water and drink as an infusion or added to green juice. I love the bitter leaves in a salad, or sautéed. — *Use in the form of the fresh leaves or capsules*

ELDERFLOWER

The oldest human-cultivated herb, elderflower has long been employed as a beauty aid to help fade freckles and age spots. Women would use infused elderflower water to help keep their skin fair and free of blemishes. The mildly astringent nature of the flowers helps to soothe mature and dry skin. I love to use it as a toner. Simply put a handful of flowerheads into a jar and pour in boiling water, then leave to stand until cool. The flowers can then be strained out and the water kept in an airtight container in the fridge to apply to the skin. I also like to add the unsweetened essence to fizzy water for a refreshing drink. — *Use in the form of the fresh flowers, tea, essence or capsules*

FENNEL SEED

I'm constantly adding fennel seeds to dishes. Containing the antioxidant quercetin, they are useful in treating and protecting against UV damage and the signs of aging. Helping to balance the skin's natural oils, the seeds are packed with vitamins and minerals such as iron, magnesium, calcium and manganese, and are great for dry and mature skin types. Like fennel itself, the seeds are a diuretic, hence great if you're feeling bloated. — *Use in the form of the whole spice or capsules*

FIGWORT

Used to speed up the healing process of irritated or burned skin, figwort is particularly helpful in the treatment of eczema and psoriasis. I like using it as a tea – 2 teaspoons of dried figwort in a cup of boiling water. It acts as a natural diuretic, so helps to flush toxins out. It can also be used in a tincture for itchy skin and psoriasis. — *Use in the form of the dried herb, tea, capsules or tinctures (a liquid extract of the herb)*

GARLIC

This is a true all-arounder, with natural antibiotic and antiviral properties that make it excellent for treating skin infections and acne. The high antioxidant content of garlic helps protect the skin from cell damage, while the sulfur it contains helps maintain the structural integrity of the skin. Most people know to cook with garlic, but if you can stomach it, eating a raw clove will help fight most infections. If you hate the taste of garlic, then simply take a garlic supplement; the properties won't be as powerful but they'll certainly be helpful. Applying crushed garlic directly to a burn can help reduce the heat and heal the skin naturally. — *Use in the form of the fresh cloves or capsules*

GINGER

Like garlic, ginger is one of those wonder foods – it's so very good for you and has a unique taste and texture. With its natural antiseptic and cleansing properties, ginger is helpful for acne and congested skin, and can even help with pigmentation and sun damage when taken internally. I'll also chop up a bit and have it in a cup of boiling water when I have an unsettled stomach, or as a tonic to begin the day. — *Use in the form of the fresh root*

LEMONGRASS

Lemongrass has an astringent effect that helps treat oily and acne-prone skin. You can add 5–10 drops of lemongrass oil to about 1 cup of a carrier oil – such as coconut oil – to apply as a cleanser to keep pores clear. It can also be used as a mosquito repellent. — *Use in the form of the fresh herb or oil*

MINT

Mint is one of my personal favorites. I always have it on hand – either in an herb box on my windowsill or in a big bunch in the fridge – for use in teas and juices. I add it to virtually any salad you care to name and it is great with chocolate too. The high levels of salicylic acid in mint make it a natural exfoliator and acne treatment, with excellent calming properties. Using mint in a fresh green juice is a super-refreshing way to start the day and I love that it's working as a sort of internal exfoliator. Mint also helps to relieve bloating by relaxing the gut wall, which helps with overall digestion. Try infusing a handful of the fresh leaves in hot water with caraway and fennel seeds as a tummy tea. You can make a toner using fresh mint (as a variant of the rosewater on p. 243). — *Use in the form of the fresh herb or tea*

NUTMEG

Nutmeg is a really warming spice, lovely for when the weather turns chillier. The spice has powerful antifungal and antibacterial properties that make it helpful for treating conditions like eczema and acne. Working to address infection on the skin, nutmeg can reduce swelling around congested pores, resulting in a smoother, clearer complexion. — *Use in the form of the ground spice*

OREGANO

For me, oregano is the flavor of Italy, where it grows freely. It has great skin-healing potential due to the antioxidant compounds that it contains – rosemarinic acid and quercetin. Known for its antibacterial properties, this herb is also antiparasitic, antiseptic and antiviral, not to mention immune-stimulating. Use in cooking or topically in the form of the essential oil, by diluting in a carrier oil and using directly. — *Use in the form of the fresh herb or oil*

PARSLEY

Parsley is excellent for balancing excess sebum secretion (oiliness) in skin, and further helps to clear congestion of the pores. The herb is packed with minerals and vitamins, while its high antioxidant content helps protect the skin from free-radical damage and helps delay the signs of aging. Use parsley just as it is to get the most out of it. If you do like the taste, parsley makes a wonderfully refreshing and healthy tea.
— *Use in the form of the fresh herb*

RED CLOVER

Taken as a tea (you can buy the dried flowerheads to infuse in hot water or use the ready-made teabags), red clover is an excellent natural treatment for eczema. Helping to eliminate toxins in the bloodstream and reducing inflammation, the herb can help to both soothe eczema outbreaks and to prevent them. Red clover-based creams can be really helpful; look out for them in a good health-food store. — *Use in the form of the dried flowerheads, tea, capsules or cream*

ROSEMARY

As well as a gorgeous aroma, rosemary has great healing potential. It is a good source of iron and magnesium, both of which help ward off tiredness and fatigue. It's also rich in compounds that act as antioxidants in the body, helping to address the damage caused to the skin by environmental factors. Rosemary water toner (made as rosewater – see p. 243) can be used on the skin as an astringent to help tighten pores. — *Use in the form of fresh/dried herb or oil*

TEA TREE

Both antifungal and antibacterial, the oil can be used as a tincture to treat cuts, insect bites and other skin problems when used diluted and applied topically. I mix a few drops of the essential oil into a carrier oil, such as organic almond oil, to create an antibacterial oil that's helpful for skin conditions on the body. For best results, look for a natural Australian tea tree oil.
— *Use in the form of a gel, oil or cream*

TURMERIC

Use as much turmeric as possible in your diet; it's an incredibly potent healing herb. A powerful all-arounder, turmeric is a blood purifier that reduces inflammation and helps the liver to detoxify, with additional benefits for both the skin and the digestive system. Turmeric may help reduce the symptoms of inflammation associated with psoriasis. I use it to make a liver tonic of my own. Squeeze half a lemon into coconut water, add 1 tbsp of flaxseed oil, a crushed garlic clove, some grated ginger and 1 tsp of ground turmeric. Blend together and drink it first thing. — *Use in the form of whole/ground root*

> *"We live in a world of instant gratification and quick fixes, but I am a true believer in the 'inside-out' approach to health and it is so refreshing to read such a concise book on this subject."* — **Amber Anderson,** model

SUPPLEMENTS AND SUPERFOODS

AÇAI BERRY

Containing one of the most potent sources of antioxidants, powdered açai berries are amazing for skin health, fighting aging free radicals and helping to brighten the complexion and support collagen production.

ACTIVATED CHARCOAL

This is used medicinally as well as in air and water purifiers. You can buy water bottles with a charcoal stick inside. The charcoal absorbs most organic toxins and harmful chemicals, and while the powder can be messy to use, it's well worth it. I use it to whiten my teeth: just use a little bit of toothpaste then dip the brush in the charcoal powder and brush. Your mouth will be black but the whitening and cleansing effect is better than any commercial product.

APPLE CIDER VINEGAR

Raw, organic, unpasteurized apple cider vinegar aids digestion by stimulating stomach acids, promoting the healthy intestinal flora and balancing the body's pH. It can be taken either neat (1 tbsp) or diluted in water.

BEE POLLEN

As bee pollen is created by worker bees to feed younger bees, it contains a wide range of vitamins and minerals to help them grow, making it a powerful superfood. It injects new life into dry skin cells and helps it look younger and more radiant. It can help to treat skin conditions like acne, eczema and almost any inflammation-based issue. It's not suitable for people with a pollen allergy.

BENTONITE CLAY

Bentonite clay is actually sourced from volcanic ash and is hugely beneficial on the whole. It can be used topically as a face mask – drawing out impurities, preventing breakouts and leaving skin baby-smooth – or you can drink it and it works in the same way to help rid the body of toxins. I add mine to smoothies to help keep my gut and skin clear.

CHIA SEED

Chia seeds are touted as a miracle food, as the vitamins, minerals and nutrients they contain are great for skin regeneration. A good source of omega-3 and omega-6 oils, as well as a complete protein, they work to build and repair tissues and help the skin to glow.

FLAXSEED

Flaxseeds are a rich, plant-based source of essential fatty acids, protein, dietary fiber, vitamins and minerals. The omega-3 and anti-inflammatory plant compounds in flaxseed promote the healing of eczema, psoriasis and acne. They're also brilliant as a natural laxative, helping the body to eliminate toxins.

HEMP SEED

These contain a good balance of omega-6 and omega-3 fatty acids, protein and vitamins (A, D and E, and many of the B-complex vitamins). Rich in sodium, calcium, iron and dietary fiber, hemp is also good for clearing up skin disorders such as psoriasis, eczema and dry skin patches. Use it instead of olive oil on a salad. This needs to be cold and so isn't suitable for cooking.

KOMBUCHA

An ancient fermented tea, kombucha encourages the growth of beneficial bacteria in the gut and helps to keep skin clear and youthful. It works to remove heavy metals and a wide range of other toxins from your body, thus keeping the skin clear and breakout-free. It improves the elasticity of your skin, along with the tone and color, acts as an internal moisturizer, and can be used as a dietary treatment for psoriasis, eczema and acne.

MANUKA HONEY

Produced in New Zealand by bees that pollinate the native manuka bush, manuka honey has great healing potential thanks to its natural antibacterial properties. Believed to address a range of stubborn "bad" bacteria and viruses in the gut, it can be used to help the skin stay clear and the body healthy. Manuka honey can also be used topically to treat acne; a potent anti-inflammatory, it soothes inflamed skin and can calm even the most chronic of skin infections. It also helps balance the skin's pH to slough away dead skin cells, enabling pores to remain clear and calming any inflammation. Apply a thin layer to your face, like a face mask, and leave it on for 5 minutes before washing off. Look for good-quality honey from a health-food store or online.

PUMPKIN SEED

Pumpkin seeds are little nutritional powerhouses – a rich source of vitamin E, zinc and omega-3 and 6 fatty acids, all of which are so beneficial for the skin and to help treat serious skin conditions. They're also said to support good gut bacteria and to rid the body of parasites. I buy them raw and organic from health-food stores and always keep the actual seeds when I cut up a pumpkin.

SPIRULINA

Known as one of the world's most nutrient-dense superfoods, spirulina is a miracle food for the skin. Loaded with proteins, vitamins (especially vitamins A, B12 and E), minerals and fatty acids, spirulina is prized for its ability to treat aging skin and dark circles under the eyes, plus it's a powerful detoxifier too. Use it in green juices for a hit of extra nutrients or see my recipe for a spirulina face mask (p. 232) to see how it can work topically on the skin, too.

WHEATGRASS

Wheatgrass juice is known for its ability to detoxify the body, helping to treat skin conditions such as acne and psoriasis, as well as addressing the signs of aging, helping to tighten loose and sagging skin and increase elasticity. Other health benefits include limiting free-radical oxidation, increasing energy, balancing blood-sugar levels, detoxifying the liver, cleansing the blood and increasing red blood cell count. A true superfood!

Dietary fiber

A well-running gut is the bedrock for good health and to achieve this, dietary fiber is essential. — *Good food sources: brown rice, pearl barley, black-eyed peas, chickpeas*

PECTIN
A form of soluble fiber, pectin aids digestion and helps lower cholesterol. — *Good food sources: apples, beets, lemons, oranges*

PREBIOTICS
Certain foods also contain non-digestible fibers that help bacteria in the gut to flourish. The fiber in these foods is often referred to as "prebiotics." — *Good food sources: bananas, garlic, Jerusalem artichokes, onions*

Fatty acids

Fat in the diet is essential for the body to work normally. Its role is to store energy, provide insulation and protect vital organs. It also produces hormones and is required for the absorption of fat-soluble vitamins from food, such as A, D, E and K. Fats are made up of fatty acids, of which there are two main types, saturated and unsaturated. Monounsaturated fats, which can be made in the body, are often considered to be the healthiest types of fat, of especial benefit to the heart. Polyunsaturated fats, also vital for health, are known as "essential fatty acids" as they can be obtained only from the diet.

OMEGA-3 AND OMEGA-6 FATTY ACIDS
These are both polyunsaturated fats. Using extra-virgin olive and coconut oil in your cooking, avoiding processed foods where possible and eating mostly plant-based foods is the best way to help maintain a good ratio of these two fatty acids in your diet. — *Good food sources: kale, sardines, tofu, walnuts*

OMEGA-9 FATTY ACIDS
One of the main monounsaturated fatty acids it has been shown to have a positive effect on cholesterol. — *Good food sources: avocados*

Minerals

Found in all foods, minerals are essential nutrients that the body requires to carry out its normal functions. Maintaining healthy bones and teeth, energy, metabolism, as well as nerve and muscle function are just a few areas of health where minerals are required.

CALCIUM
Vital for healthy bones and teeth, and important for muscle function, blood pressure and the heart. It also helps to regulate skin cell production and repair. — *Good food sources: sardines, sesame seeds, tofu*

CHROMIUM
Helps to regulate blood-sugar levels and to reduce spikes, which may age the skin, and to curb sugar cravings. — *Good food sources: asparagus, bananas, beef, mushrooms*

COPPER
Essential for the condition of the skin, by repairing and maintaining connective tissue. — *Good food sources: chickpeas, miso, kale*

IODINE
Essential for a healthy thyroid gland, one of whose key roles is to regulate the metabolism, which impacts on weight levels. — *Good food sources: eggs, salmon, sardines, seaweed*

IRON

Essential for the production of healthy red blood cells. Low levels – particularly common among women – can lead to tiredness and fatigue as well as dry hair and skin. — *Good food sources: eggs, beef, kale, dark chocolate*

MAGNESIUM

A stress-busting nutrient, magnesium helps to reduce stress and relax muscles, helping with sleep quality as a result. — *Good food sources: bananas, brown rice, kale, quinoa*

MANGANESE

Helps to promote elasticity and aid in repair. — *Good food sources: brown rice, chickpeas, walnuts, quinoa, spinach, tofu*

PHOSPHORUS

A general immune system booster. — *Good food sources: beef, leeks, white fish, tomatoes*

POTASSIUM

Helps to control the balance of fluids in the body and is required for proper nerve and muscle function. — *Good food sources: mushrooms, pumpkins, salmon, zucchini*

SELENIUM

A great help for the skin, this antioxidant helps to protect against and repair UV damage. — *Good food sources: eggs, pearl barley, chicken, spinach*

SILICA

Silica activates enzymes involved in the production of collagen. — *Good food sources: cucumber, leeks, rhubarb, strawberries*

SULFUR

Helps support the connective tissue and collagen for firmer, younger-looking skin. — *Good food sources: garlic, onions*

ZINC

Helps to regulate over 200 hormones, including testosterone. — *Good food sources: chicken, dark chocolate, sesame seeds*

Phytochemicals

These are compounds found in plants, and although not essential to health they do provide additional protection against disease.

CAROTENOIDS

This group of compounds help to reduce inflammation, while the carotenes (alpha and beta) can be converted to vitamin A (see below) in the body, which is essential for cell repair and renewal. — *Good food sources: leafy greens, avocados, egg, watermelon*

FLAVONOIDS

Flavonoids are a group of plant chemicals that have been shown to help reduce the risk of disease in the body. They behave as powerful antioxidants and help to fight-free radical damage. — *Good food sources: eggplant, pomegranates, strawberries*

GLUTATHIONE

A powerful antioxidant that aids the skin by boosting its detoxification processes, and by strengthening the immune system. — *Good food sources: apples, asparagus, avocados, bananas, beets, carrots*

POLYPHENOLS

Antioxidant compounds that help to reduce the risk of disease. — *Good food sources: dark chocolate, natural red wine, oranges, pomegranates, white tea*

Probiotics

Probiotics (see also p. 14) are live bacteria that can be found in foods and help to maintain a healthy gut. — *Good food sources: kefir, Greek yogurt, miso*

Protein

The role of protein in the body is for the repair and maintenance of your body's tissues. — *Good vegetarian food sources: alfalfa sprouts, eggs, quinoa, tofu, pearl barley*

Vitamins

VITAMIN A
Helps to slow the aging process – essential for cell repair and renewal, and cell turnover too. — *Good food sources: eggs, carrots, kale, pumpkins, tomatoes*

B1 (THIAMINE)
Helps to support the nervous system, energy levels and digestive function. — *Good food sources: avocados, eggs, kale, spinach*

B2 (RIBOFLAVIN)
Essential for healthy hair and nails as well as skin. — *Good food sources: asparagus, eggs, mushrooms, sesame seeds*

B3 (NIACIN)
Maintains good circulation. — *Good food sources: avocados, chicken, eggs*

B5 (PANTOTHENIC ACID)
Promotes moisturization of the skin. — *Good food sources: brown rice, eggs, quinoa*

B6 (PYRIDOXINE)
Great support for mood, regulates sleep and a healthy immune system. — *Good food sources: avocados, bananas, chicken, garlic*

B7 (BIOTIN)
Supports the adrenal system, regulates metabolism and helps maintain healthy skin, hair and nails. — *Good food sources: brown rice, eggs*

B9 (FOLATE)
Repairs skin cells. — *Good food sources: avocados, black-eyed peas, carrots, chickpeas, eggs, spinach*

B12 (COBALAMIN)
Boosts energy levels. — *Good food sources: eggs, sardines, seaweed*

CHOLINE
Helps maintain a healthy metabolism. — *Good food sources: eggs, salmon*

VITAMIN C (ASCORBIC ACID)
Promotes collagen production and improves elasticity for more toned-looking skin. — *Good food sources: lemons, oranges, kiwi fruit, pomegranates, pumpkins, radishes, spinach*

VITAMIN D
This vitamin works to improve mood and the immune system in general, which is especially important during the winter months when there is a lack of sun. — *Good food sources: eggs, mushrooms*

VITAMIN E (ALPHA-TOCOPHEROL)
Acts as an internal moisturizer for a soft, wrinkle-free complexion. — *Good food sources: avocados, leafy greens, spinach, tomatoes*

VITAMIN K
Vitamin K helps the blood to clot and strengthens blood vessels, thus reducing the appearance of dark circles under the eyes and helping to prevent varicose veins. — *Good food sources: asparagus, avocados, beets, kale, parsley, red cabbage, spinach*

ACKNOWLEDGMENTS

Did I ever think it could be like this? No I didn't. Did I ever think I was going to write a book? No, that's for sure, being dyslexic and having only read five books in my life, I'm honestly much better at looking at pictures. I'm far too impatient to concentrate on one thing for too long, with books I usually dip in and out.

That being said, I need to thank all these people because without them this wouldn't have been possible.

Caren Fisk, my agent and lifelong friend, for supporting me throughout the years through the really shitty times and great times too, for always being constant and never changing our focus, and for believing in me even if I didn't.

Charlotte Ridge and Adrian Sington for the initial idea and for believing that I could do this.

Jessica Clark, for the immense amount of research you did in the shortest amount of time possible. For giving me the backbone of the book, I couldn't have done it without you. All my love.

David Loftus and Frankie Unsworth, my newfound friends, for allowing me to be the art director, on and off site, for forgiving all my faux pas, like directing from another photo shoot over the phone and standing in the kitchen and generally just getting in the way. Who do I think I am, Anna Wintour? Thank you for your patience and for the amazing images; they are everything and more than I expected.

Camilla for your support, energy, enthusiasm, thoughtfulness and of course for the beautiful images. I couldn't have done it without you. For always bringing it back to basics – as you always like to go on about. This time it was on our shoot, arriving like gypsies – styling, props, and art direction. Thank you for allowing me to put the pressure on by trying to fit every shoot we've done in the last ten years into one day. A heart-felt thanks! Big love to your agent Karin Lund for making it all work.

I've never met a person like Kate Parker, my copy editor, a person with ultimate patience and who can remember every part of a book – I couldn't and I wrote it! Thank you.

My oldest friends, Mercedes Gutierrez and Elliott Smedley, thank you for putting up with me, listening to my rants, my know-all-ness and ideas. All the words of wisdom, for your inspiration and style, and all the sidesplitting laughter. Mercedes, for always being my sounding board and keeping things in perspective. Elliott for being that grounding force, even though sometimes I don't want to hear it. I love you both dearly.

Jem Mitchell, for being so accommodating and a constant support, always taking great portraits and adding to my collages, thank you so much.

Earl Simms, for the years of friendship and giving me your secret recipe, for being a hilarious sous chef and cooking buddy who says he's not helping but can't stop nosing around the kitchen. Thank you for being a constant form of entertainment. Big love.

Ali Pirzadeh (hairdresser) for being so accommodating to make this work and your willingness to come along for the ride.

Ben Jones, for your generosity and helping me add to this book. Big kiss.

Dom Harlow, for being a great cooking teammate, for our signature dishes, for your precise recipes and swift replies. Natasha and Patrick Graeme-Baker, for cooking from afar and for being so generous with your time and expertise. Thanks to Jethro Turner.

To my dear friend Sienna Miller, for writing my foreword and being so excited that I asked you; you always blow me away with your humility, even when you remind me that we're not the same age! And also thanks to Tori Cook.

Anja Rubik, for allowing me to use beautiful images and giving me her support, for her tasting and input, and for generally being a great friend. Toni Garrn, thanks for being super funny always! Love our images. Victoria Beckham for always loving what I do and supporting me. And also thanks to Natalie Lewis too.

The beautiful model Tuva Alfredsson for being so generous.

Sienna King, I always love working with you – such a happy soul to be around and such an amazing face.

Gladys Brown – really great to meet you by chance; thank you for helping me create beautiful images.

Neelam Gill, thank you for your beautiful spirit and kind words. Suki Waterhouse, for your kooky spin on stuff, I love it! Amber Anderson, for being so supportive and generally a lovely person. Cara Delevingne, for being part of my journey. Kathy Phillips for your like-minded approach to beauty. Christopher Bailey, CEO of Burberry, for your belief in me and all your years of support.

To Holly Star – thank you for your guidance and helping me to get to this point. Looking forward to future endeavours. Lots of love . . . Namaste.

A big thanks to the team at Random House: Lizzy Gray, Clarissa Pabi, Sarah Bennie, Lisa Dyer and Helen Everson. Especially to Louise McKeever. Rob Hobson, for your knowledge. Sandra Zellmer for the beautiful book design. My food tasters Tim Howard, Aliana Lopez and Mark.

I just have to say this was a journey and this was the final piece of this intricate puzzle. And I must say I enjoyed writing this part most! It would have been longer but I ran out of space!

Wendy x

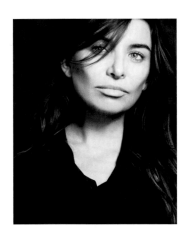

With more than twenty years
of experience working with
A-list models and celebrities,
international makeup artist
WENDY ROWE is known
for her uncomplicated and
holistic approach to skincare.
She is Burberry's artistic
consultant to beauty.

www.wendyrowe.com

 @wendyrowemakeup

 @wendyrowe